Why Children Don't Listen

119

Why Children Don't Listen

A Guide for Parents and Teachers

Monika Kiel-Hinrichsen

Floris Books

Translated by Anna Cardwell

First published in German in 2005
under the title *Warum Kinder nicht zuhören*
by Verlag Freies Geistesleben & Urachhaus GmbH, Stuttgart
First published in English in 2006 by Floris Books, Edinburgh

© 2005 Verlag Freies Geistesleben & Urachhaus GmbH, Stuttgart
This translation © 2006 Floris Books, Edinburgh

British Library CIP Data available

ISBN-10 0-86315-574-X
ISBN-13 978-086315-574-1

Printed in Great Britain
by Bell & Bain, Glasgow

Contents

Foreword   9

1. What is the Aim of this Book?   11
   What this book does not want to do   12

2. Listen to What I Say   15
   Insights into day-to-day life   15

3. The Process of Childhood   21
   The development of the child in the first seven years   21
   The development of the school child
       from seven to fourteen years   26
   Puberty from fourteen to twenty-one years   31
       Intellectual puberty   32
       Emotional puberty   34
       Will puberty   34

4. It is Only With the Heart that One Can See Rightly   37
   Fine tuning the instrument of the soul   39
       Looking into the heart of the child   41

5. Speak, and You Reveal Yourself   43
   Body language, soul language   43
   The meaning of the voice for educating hearing   47
       Exercises for partner or parent's groups   49

6. Speaking, Listening, Understanding   53
   Sending four messages   54
   Receiving with four ears   56

7. Transaction Analysis and Bringing up Children   61
   Parents, children and adults in one person   61
   The Parent Ego State   61
   The Adult Ego State   63
   The Child Ego State   63
   The development of personality parts   65
       Up until six months of age   65
       From six to eighteen months   67

From eighteen to thirty-six months 68
From three to six years 70
From six to twelve years 72
From thirteen to nineteen years 74
*Empathy exercises to help understand
the child's personality parts* 77
The four fundamental life attitudes 80
Basic transaction patterns 82
Complementary transactions 83
Crossed transactions 85
Covert transactions 87
Transactions in day-to-day family life 88

8. Education Towards a 'Whole Human Being' 93
Education of the senses and social abilities 93
Introduction to the teaching of the senses 95
The four lower senses, basal sense, will sense 95
*The four central senses — environmental senses —
sensation senses* 98
Lack of sense experiences and their compensation 104
What does the development of the senses
have to do with the ability to listen? 108
ADHD children and hearing 109
*Suggestions and exercises for training
children's twelve senses* 111

9. The Competence of Today's Children 117
Aggressiveness as a warning sign 120
Aggression creates meetings 121
Aggression: an open dam 122
From frustration to aggression 123
Emotional intelligence as the basis for competence 126
Exercise questions for creating emotional competence 130

10. From Upbringing to a Relationship 131
The five basic needs of the human being 134
Exercise for the five basic needs of the human being 137
Needs have to be taken seriously 138
About the art of listening 140
Educating towards conflict ability 143
Active listening; from you-messages to I-messages 143
Exercises for sending I-messages 149

11. Family Conflict Management   153
    The family conference   153
    If it is not so easy to solve   156

12. Self-discipline as the Basis of Bringing up Children   161
    Getting to know your inner team   161
    Five phases of inner conflict management   164
    Soul hygiene as the basis for a new perception   165
       Subsidiary exercises of Rudolf Steiner   166

13. Psychological Distress and the Birth Pangs of the
    Consciousness Soul   175

    Endnotes   181
    Bibliography   185

'If you want a friend, tame me!'
'What must I do to tame you?' asked the little prince.
'You must be very patient,' replied the fox.
'First you will sit down in the grass at a little distance from me. I shall look at you out of the corner of my eye, and you will say nothing. Words are the source of misunderstandings. But every day, you will be able to sit a little closer to me.'

Antoine de Saint-Exupéry, *The Little Prince*

Foreword

Monika Kiel-Hinrichsen writes at the end of this book that the actual title should be 'It is only with the heart that one can see rightly.' With this book she would like to contribute towards a practical teaching of life and soul. The title is now directed more towards the child: *Why children don't listen,* or asked as a question: *Why don't children listen?* This book makes it clear that children want to show us adults that the question needs to be asked in a different way if we want to receive a truly human answer. First of all Monika Kiel-Hinrichsen poses the question about our own capacity to listen. 'Am I capable of listening to the child?' We are encouraged to open ourselves up towards the other person and become more self-aware. Many exercises and suggestions help us to achieve this goal. Am I able to make space in my soul for my child to express itself, for it to be heard? Somewhere where I do not only hear the words, but also understand the message conveyed both by words and other verbal gestures. My capacity to 'listen beyond the words' is related to my willingness and ability to create a silence within myself. This silence cannot come about without conscious effort, as the soul notices all possible and impossible things. An intimate, completely individual I-force, revealed in everyday life through modesty, enables this silence to enter into the soul. I make myself capable of listening with the innermost part of my soul, and because of this am able to perceive what is essential in the other person, in the child.

Practise the exercises in this book using this kind of I-force! Find out which ones are most important for you. You will need to 'individualize' the exercises, then something deeply human, and also practical, can occur.

This book will help parents and children form a closer relationship with each other. Particularly in this time of psychological distress they have a lot to teach each other. Monika Kiel-Hinrichsen deserves our thanks; from her own experience she hands us a key to open the door to the inner space for listening.

Paul Mackay
Leader of the Section for Social Sciences at the
Goetheanum, Dornach, Switzerland

1. What is the Aim of this Book?

During the course of my pedagogical work, educational counselling, as well as bringing up my own children I was repeatedly
confronted with questions and phenomena related to speaking,
listening and understanding. Parents, mainly mothers, come for
educational advice or to parental supervision groups because
they feel overwhelmed by the task of bringing up children.
Children listen increasingly less to what their parents say; they
do what they want, let messages go in one ear and out the other,
and defy their parents.

Six years ago with this fact in mind the speech therapist,
Andreas Voigt, and I started giving seminars with the title:
'Speak so I can hear you.' The title was put from the child's
point of view and directed with eye and ear towards the
parents: how should I speak as a mother/father or teacher
so that it is 'worth' the child's while to listen to me, so that
I am heard? Characteristically, a mother called to enrol and
formulated the title in the opposite way: 'I would like to take
part in the seminar "Listen to what I say."' I had to laugh
heartily.

In the seminars, but also on playgrounds, on the beach, in
shopping centres etc I have noticed how much insecurity parents
radiate when dealing with their children. How little clarity and
certainty is expressed linguistically. Often a sentence, which is
meant as a command, sounds like a question. 'Now tidy up your
room, okay?' — the voice pitch rises at the end of the sentence.
One can often see the resulting insecurity on the child's face.
And the view inside the child's mind is: Mummy said I should
tidy up, but I can decide if it's okay or not. So I'll say no!

Or the question: 'Shall we go now?' Usually this means: 'I
want to go now' — 'No, not yet!' — 'But I want to, we'll go in
five minutes!'

It is a definite fact that deep in their hearts all parents only want the best for their child. Usually they would like to do a better job than their own parents, and attempt to create a relationship based on partnership. Children are given a say in the matter, but parents are not able to subsequently carry this partnership through as, naturally, children cannot make all the decisions. This leads to the more powerful one winning, although it is often not clear where the power and where the powerlessness lies. The small sentence appendage 'okay?' opens the door for discussions between parents and children, which often end in exhaustion, annoyance and aggression. And then speech begins to have a different effect as the stronger the feelings that are aroused, the more confusing the messages that parents send and children pick up.

Many conflicts could be avoided if we paid more attention to our own thinking, feelings, actions and speech. This is what this book aims to encourage. It aims to draw attention to deep-seated habits, which express themselves through body language with all its nuances. It wants to give the reader courage to go on a soul-excursion and get to know the 'inner child' and the 'inner parents,' or the 'inner team,' to bring greater clarity into upbringing. The exercises also invite you to do this. These have almost all been tested for their effectiveness through personal experience and parent work. Look on them as suggestions to be personally adapted. Have fun!

What this book does not want to do:
The content of this book is not supposed to give parents a guilty conscience or feelings of incompetence, but help them to rethink and work through old patterns and structures. Parents are not superhuman, who can react trained and competent at all times, for that the task of upbringing is too all-encompassing and the distance we usually have in our normal work life from our tasks, which enable a relatively objective point of view, does not exist for parents. The suggestions using the communication models should not be understood to be present at all times.

Instead, a healthy row, also called 'holy anger' by Rudolf Steiner, can achieve miracles and can have a noticeable 'cleansing' effect on upbringing.

My thanks go to the many parents that gave me their trust in the different courses. A good question already carries part of the answer in it, in this sense I was also able to receive a lot from the parents. Special thanks goes to Christiane Unrau who, as mother of four children, tested the contents of this book for its usefulness in day-to-day life. I would also like to thank my patient family, who did without me for many an hour while I was writing this book and who supported me sympathetically.

2. Listen to What I Say

Insights into day-to-day life

Josefa is on the phone, trying desperately to keep track of the conversation with her friend. 'Mummy,' the four and a half-year-old Antonella keeps interrupting, 'I want to go to kindergarten!' — 'Soon, Antonella — go and brush your teeth and put your shoes on.' But nothing happens! Josefa continues speaking on the phone, sometimes gesticulating with annoyance towards her daughter, who in turn is crouched on the floor and keeps interrupting her mother's conversation. The situation escalates. Josefa becomes angry, breaks off the conversation with her friend, as she could not solve her problem like this on the telephone, and turns to Antonella reproachfully. 'You always disturb me when I'm phoning, you could've easily brushed your teeth, now we'll be late for kindergarten!' At the same time she thinks of her friend with annoyance, who keeps phoning her early in the morning with her problems. Antonella becomes obstinate, she starts to kick her boots through the hallway and hit Josefa. 'Now stop it,' Josefa shouts, 'You never listen to what I say!' She takes Antonella's hand forcefully and goes to the bathroom with her. Reluctantly the latter starts cleaning her teeth.

Josefa feels exhausted and close to tears. She watches her daughter in the mirror cleaning her teeth and slowly feelings of guilt begin to stir in her, Josefa starts an inner dialogue: how often have I resolved not to answer the phone if I haven't got time to talk anyway? — Yes, but surely it is possible to exchange a few sentences, Antonella is old enough to ... No, she isn't. I had resolved to do everything in peace, to give her some attention in the morning. But at least she could have cleaned her teeth by herself!

Meanwhile, Antonella is finished and ready to go to kindergarten, she happily warbles a song to herself and everything seems forgotten.

Susan's family is a different case. Susan is the mother of two sons aged ten and fourteen, and is a single working mother. Susan is sitting at the table reading the daily newspaper, it is late afternoon, and all she wants to do is drink her coffee in peace. The door opens and her ten-year-old son, Matthew, enters. Joyfully he tells her about the bicycle test he has passed. Susan looks up tiredly from reading the newspaper. 'How nice for you,' and then continues reading. Disappointedly Matthew goes into his room, turns on his tape recorder and thinks to himself: Stupid mum, I revised for so long and all she says is 'how nice for you,' everything is stupid at home.

A little later John crashes into the house and flops into an armchair; he looks pale and over-fatigued. Susan looks up: 'Hallo, how are you?' John starts talking about a conflict with his class teacher but Susan is already absorbed in her newspaper. He gets up, goes to his room and lies down on his bed.

Two hours later all three of them meet again at the supper table. Susan is annoyed that none of the chores have been done, she criticizes the boys. Susan also starts an inner dialogue: everybody here does exactly what he or she wants. Nobody is responsible for the community. It's actually all too much for me! She looks at her two sons accusingly and questioningly.

John takes heart: 'We always have to do everything for you, but you're not interested at all in what we do!' Now that he's said it, the knot in Matthew's throat also loosens.

Susan becomes thoughtful and full of consternation, feels her exhaustion, her temporary inability to get involved with the boys, her longing for a partner to take some of the load off her. And she realizes how difficult she finds it to react appropriately to the children. She sees herself confronted with her old problem of withdrawing and 'shielding' herself.

I myself experienced a situation with my eldest daughter recently that made me feel ashamed as I felt unexpectedly caught out. After a strenuous day I wanted to be alone in the sitting room, but she was sitting there listening to music and reading. When I asked her if she didn't have to revise for her exams, I received the irritated answer: 'Do you want me to leave?' How right she was!

I believe the situations described above are normal day-to-day family conflicts familiar to most of us. In family life with all its different obligations we especially need a high level of receptiveness and perceptiveness. But where can we receive energy and inspiration when struggling for these qualities in bringing up children or in social relationships in general? How can I acquire the necessary 'presence of mind' at the right time, or deal with 'conflict management' in the family?

For many *children* upbringing often means: prohibitions, commands and accusations. These cause an unstoppable chain reaction in the form of resistance.

Many *parents* feel overburdened by the task of bringing up children, which they are not able to deal with simply because they have become parents. Any other job includes training, but in a certain sense one is thrown into being a parent without any previous preparation. So what can be the basis for bringing up kids?

In many cases, and this is confirmed by my knowledge in biographical counselling, it is not the experiences one has with one's own parents. One wants to do it better than them! Prior to becoming parents people study psychological and pedagogical books, which reveal good intentions to do it differently, with more consciousness. Probably you, dear readers, have taken this book to hand for these reasons. But, despite the best intentions, the moment comes when the children succeed in pushing you to your limits, and the eighties quote from the author, Nancy Friday, becomes reality: 'I look into the mirror and see my mother,' or in the spirit of emancipation: 'I look into the mirror and see my father.' We discover values and behavioural patterns that we thought we had overcome years ago. Characteristically, the mother of a three-year-old child in one of the seminars once expressed this with the words: 'I never thought that a young child would be capable of bringing out my darker side!' She then described the moments when she suddenly screamed at her child, gave him a slap on the backside or sent him to his room as a punishment.

Which phenomena exist when such regressive steps in our development happen?

A new phase in life starts for most people with a first pregnancy, particularly for the mother, which is comparable to a journey in a small, often lonely boat drifting on still unknown waters without real control or the knowledge of navigation. Only slowly does one learn to take the oars in hand and become more confident. At the same time one may glance at the shores occasionally, to the place where there was still a certain freedom, self-certainty and recognition through ones work before the family was started. In those days there was still free time to recuperate, for example, sufficient sleep, time for cultural interests and, above all, time to spend together with your partner. I particularly want to mention these privileges, the lack of which often leads to tension or even full-blown conflict in family life, which then lead to identity crises:

• Who am I? Which role do I fulfil? (mother/father/
  partner);
• How am I a mother/father/partner?
• How do I want to bring up my child?

The circumstances described above bring parents back into old behavioural patterns as exhaustion, stress and extreme demands reawaken old connections in the brain, experienced during childhood, which now shape our behaviour. This does not mean we are trapped in a dead end without escape. It is exactly this awakening process that motivates us to take the next step. In his book the neurobiologist, Gerald Hüther, describes access routes, developmental paths, dead ends, ways out and new ways.[1] I aim to contribute to the new ways in the sense of the words 'It is only with the heart that one can see rightly.'

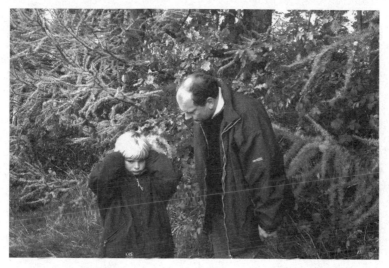

Everyone has probably experienced or observed a moment like this: Although the educator is trying hard to have a conflict free conversation, the situation suddenly gets out of hand and the child refuses all cooperation.

Through my own experiences as a mother, but also through my experiences with pedagogical work and counselling I would like to attempt to introduce you, the reader, to different areas and options of working through conflicts, starting from the anthroposophical study of the human being. This premeditates becoming familiar with the stages of development of the child, as communication can be expanded and made more conscious when taking developmental stages into account.

3. The Process of Childhood

I would like to address your 'adult Ego State' in this chapter. You can find out more about this in the following chapters. But for now I will only explain this much: We process information with our adult Ego State and obtain an overview in thinking, which in turn helps us to achieve an objective stance out of our subjective affectedness. Everything that is lifted into our consciousness brings us further along the path to inner freedom.

Gaining a rudimentary understanding of the developmental phases of children is a good foundation and creates the space for social working together, for communication.

The development of the child in the first seven years

Within the first year of life the inner activity of the child turns towards the outside world and the discovery of its own physical body. If we follow this process attentively, then we can see that to start with the own body of the child is still a small 'outer world.'. The child discovers his little hands moving across his field of vision and uses them as a first toy, then he finds his legs and feet, sucks his big toe, and suddenly everything disappears from view again. Once the child has discovered his body and learnt to control it to some extent he starts to straighten up from the horizontal position, finds a new orientation in space and grasps and experiences it in three dimensions by crawling and standing up. Soon the child takes his first step and a small human ready for action stands before us.

This process of standing up is the first actual human expression after smiling. The small person learns to stand up and walk by imitating his surroundings. Each child has his own characteristic way of learning to stand up. One child sits for a long time and only crawls a bit, while another one crawls swiftly around, suddenly pulls himself up and walks off courageously. During this process one can already observe the different temperaments of the children and receive indications of the developing personality.

Once the toddler has learnt to walk he starts detaching himself from the close relationship with his mother and begins to widen his sphere of action. Now a new typically human ability starts to develop — speech. Previously the toddler has tried out all kinds of sounds, in a certain sense he has 'felt' his way into the sounds, as well as listening to those from his parents and his surroundings. The small child is still receptive to all the fine tones and emotional undertones of the speaker and reacts to emotional nuances.

> 'It orientates and orders itself on the I activity
> of its surroundings, which are expressed through
> speech, and thus it receives the necessary forces
> for its incarnation [...] We can clearly see how
> the initially unformed [...] voice material is
> worked on [...] how the soul of the child man-
> ages to take hold of the body more and more
> strongly, until — around the third year — the
> I itself articulates itself, if still in a dreamlike-
> unconscious way.'[2]

With these forces the child now starts to develop his speech through movement. He starts to speak whole words, and while he practises walking, skipping and jumping his speech is also organized into sentence structure and tenses.

The development of thinking is directly related to walking and talking — and with it perception awakens. The child has conquered part of the spatial outer world. The very first kind of memory occurs. Bit by bit the soul has worked its way into the body and made it into a tool for the 'I.' This moment can be seen when the child stops calling himself by his first name and starts experiencing and calling himself an 'I.'

When the child learns to articulate during his third year he becomes increasingly 'organized.' The initially twitchy, restless soul of the child starts to become more peaceful.[3] But he also has an increasing desire to experience himself through his personality. Up until this point he was a 'being of impressions,' a being of the senses on which the outer world had left an impression, now he becomes an expressive person, someone who wishes to express himself. And how does the child do this? By showing that he wants to go his own way, that he wants to sense itself. This is when the terrible twos begin — a time full of conflict, which can lead to communication disturbances between parent and child. The obstinate child often pushes his parents to the limits of their loving behaviour. The awakening I of the child becomes a target for parents to increasingly give commands and prohibitions, as well as criticism. I compiled the following list of commands and prohibitions, which most children hear countless times, in my book *Why children are obstinate:*[4]

COMMANDS	PROHIBITIONS
Sit still.	Don't touch that.
Clean your teeth.	Don't fall into the water.
Put your slippers on.	Don't climb up there.
Leave that alone.	Don't tease your sister.
Come here.	Don't spill it.
Stand still.	Don't make a mess.
Eat up.	Don't dawdle.
Leave me in peace.	Don't shout so loudly
Be quiet.	Don't walk away.
Stop picking your nose.	Don't hit your sister.
Say hello.	Don't get dirty.
Come and eat.	Don't wet your pants.

In a seminar, one of the fathers took stock of this jokingly and said: 'Be different.'

If we think of all these commands and prohibitions in relation to ourselves — for example, from a continually fault-finding partner, then we can easily empathize with the feelings of the child. Instead of feeling seen or accepted inside, we would feel challenged to resist or refuse. The defiant child is doing nothing else. He protects himself through defiance.

At the same the small child consciously starts examining the outer world. he experiences himself as an I with recently awakened conscious forces, but in fact these forces still come from a dream land. With his senses and will power, and less with abstract thinking, he is devoted to the surroundings. The child's imitative being orientates him completely to using adults as his example.

Four great maxims are the cornerstones of bringing up children in their first seven years of life:

> *Example and imitation,*
> *Rhythm and repetition.*

The small child wants us to speak to him in such a way that he can be an imitator. If, from an early age, he lives in a creative surrounding structured by rhythm, then good habits are formed which avoid correction in other situations.

During this stage the child begins to be stimulated by the fundamental nature of his direct surroundings; he becomes a creator using his wonderful gift of imagination, which awakens around the end of his third year and enables the child to discover his surroundings with increasingly creative play. Now he is able to transform a table into a house or a ship. A building block can become an animal, a cloth becomes water or a meadow. Imagination and images filled with truth are his soul's building blocks for the creation of his world. In contrast, clearly outlined concepts and abstract explanations bounce off the child, and turn him into a being of resistance.

In this context Rudolf Steiner reminds us that a child up to his fifth year has no sense of what it should do, but is a will person. This gives rise to the pedagogical question: How can the child voluntarily do what he is supposed to do?

Example: *Mary, four and a half years old, is deeply engrossed playing with her dolls; she is dressing them up as they are going to a party. It is late and Mary's mother is getting impatient. She admonishes her that it is time to go, which has no effect on Mary. Her mother knows from experience that there will be tears if she takes Mary away from her play. So she tries to connect with Mary's play and takes the little doll's suitcase with the words: 'Mary, you need to pack the suitcase quickly, the train is about to leave.' Meanwhile, she herself also packs the necessary things, including a small snack. — In this way Mary does not really feel disturbed, her emotions are included in her mother's intentions.*

Between the fifth and sixth year, increasing insight and understanding leads to a different will quality in the child, which can also be called goal-orientated. The child is not satisfied solely with his creative imagination, but wants this to be related to reality. While formerly the most important aspect of building a tunnel in the sandpit was the process of building, now the goal — that a car can drive through the tunnel — becomes central The freeing up of his imaginative forces gives the child the chance to use his will towards achieving a goal. This is the transitional phase to school.

This process makes it possible to talk to the child in a different way; the child becomes able to understand relationships in the world in a different way.

Example: *Anthony is kneeling in the sandpit and is a road worker. He has a precise idea of what he wants: a bridge spanning two roads. He has collected pieces of wood, but unfortunately everything keeps falling down. First Anthony becomes angry, then he starts crying desperately. His father joins him: 'Anthony, what's wrong, is something not working? Do you need help?' Together they think of a solution. Anthony's* *father notices that Anthony needs a bit of support, although he already has an idea. He tries to help him so that Anthony is the one who finds a solution for the problem. Contentedly Anthony stands in front of his bridge, which had only needed a few skilful improvements.*

The development of the school child from seven to fourteen years

The child goes through an important change during the course of its seventh year, which is characterized physically by an incredible growth spurt and the loss of milk teeth. The child lives through a change of form. From a spiritual point of view new consciousness and imaginative forces are liberated which previously worked internally on the physical body as life-forces, giving the child his individual form. A clear sign for the end of this phase is when the second teeth break through; these are like a memorial for the formative forces of the first seven-year period. Now the child starts a first emotional transformation, which some parents already experience as a small puberty. Naturally, this is not the case, even if we can find emotional parallels.

During the seventh year the child starts distancing himself from his close parental surroundings. Just like he gained a first I-consciousness and started to construct a provisional view of the world at around the age of three, he now feels the need to portray this world-view to his surroundings and modify it through increasing world experience.

Independently he now enters a new phase of life. Formerly he was guided by parents and sustained by familiar habits, now he enters a new phase of the journey into the larger social environment. This leads to entirely independent experiences, unsettling the limited world-view of a seven year old. 'Why can't I watch TV? I want to watch …!' or 'Tim's got a game boy, and I don't!' or 'I want a magazine subscription too!' etc. A phase of separation commences, which leads to an ever-increasing sphere of action and experience. The first thin wall arises between the inner and outer world, which thickens as the child matures. We can imagine this wall as a second skin — an emotional skin. The child becomes more independent, his I-consciousness stronger, with the growth of this emotional skin.

This process does not normally proceed without irritations. The emotional conversion stands in direct relationship to physical reorganization. With the loss of his milk teeth the child looses his old face in a certain sense, he feels thrown off centre both physically and emotionally.

Thus the child needs to find a new centre. On the one hand this is formed in the mouth, when the front teeth change. The child manages to achieve centrality in the head and develops laterality, that is, he develops a sure feeling of right and left and an understanding of symmetry. This shows that one of the basic conditions for school learning has awakened.

We can observe the disharmony in the developing school child, which is also comparable to the period of obstinacy. While around the third year the I of the child is first born, around the seventh year this childhood I is strengthened.

In both phases we are dealing with untamed childhood willpower, which expresses itself in emotional disunity in the form of resistance and the need for love. The conflict between abating introversion and emerging extroversion, with which the child wants to express himself ever more strongly, lead many children to feel insecure and empty. Often the emotional changes of this life phase are expressed in the form of fear. Fear of the dark and waking from nightmares are familiar symptoms of this time.[5]

Example: *Christine lost her first milk tooth when she was five years old. The entire 'tooth change' process lasted between four and eight weeks, from the 'wobbling' of her milk tooth to the fully-grown adult tooth.*

Christine's 'emotional change' started with the wobbling of the first upper tooth (at about six and three quarters). A new person awoke from this dreamy school child, who now had to learn to cope with the world she now perceived. Often she could not stand upright on her two feet, and lay or 'sprawled' on the floor, or had to lean against something. Her speech and expressions appeared to be in a kind of 'pre-puberty' stage. We often noticed a strong disunity, expressed by loud behaviour and strong emotional outbursts and protest. She needed close physical contact and often looked for the chance to experience herself.

The conflict between 'growing up' and 'wanting to remain little' was expressed almost daily. On the one hand she wanted to decide everything herself, on the other hand she still wanted to be carried around and treated like a small child.

Rudolf Steiner describes the change of the soul-forces described above as a great 'battle state,' which occurs within the child.[6] In this phase of life the liberated ether body 'struggles' against the astral body, the growth-forces against the forces that work in the maturing breath. We have seen in the above section that with the change of teeth forces of consciousness are set free that previously worked as growth forces in the body shaping the organs. A large amount of these forces still remain in the body and cause growth until puberty, but at the same time they oppose that which occurs through the changing breathing process of the child. Up until the twelfth year the blood-breathing process has harmonized. While a toddler breathes up to twenty times as often as an adult, the breathing rhythm starts to calm down around the ninth or tenth year. This increasingly deep breathing stimulates life processes in the child, as oxygen in the blood kindles the burning in the cells, which stimulates the metabolism. A new contact between heart and lung develops, a new relationship between their rhythms, which contributes to the development of an emotional inner space in the child. A clear sign of this process is the emotional forces that appear with the deepened breathing.

Every emotion expresses itself in some way through breathing. Anger leads to heavy but blocked breathing. When happy exhalation prevails, in fear or sadness we hold our breath, and when calm we breathe deeply.

We have seen how the child-like emotions go through a process of great change during this phase of life, although the child's emotions still have to be clearly set apart from the emotional life of an adult. Up until the ninth year, feelings and the will can hardly be differentiated. It is only when the breathing starts to mature — initially around the ninth, tenth year with the ratio 1:4 (breathing: pulse) — that one can experience how children can have feelings within themselves without making them visible to the outside world through words and actions.[7] The emotions have become further removed from the direct will and physical imprisonment (as is the case in the first seven years). An increasingly independent soul-space is born which can mediate between thoughts and actions.

In this case we can speak of a further I-birth or I-incarnation, as the I connects itself to the metabolism through the harmony between breathing and pulse.[8]

Example: *Mary is just nine years old but has a choleric temperament. She has a tendency to colds when she also gets a high temperature. On the one hand she confronts parents and teachers with vehemence, on the other hand she asks for a light to be left on in the evenings and the door left ajar so that she does not get scared. While she used to remain by herself for an hour in the evening, now she refuses to. During the holidays her mother reads her a book. She identifies so strongly with a being whose crown is dirty and needs to be cleaned that she cries desperately and starts thinking about how dirty her own crown is. Her mother finds it difficult to comfort her or to understand what is happening in her.*

All these occurrences are signs of an important moment in the child's biography, as now he experiences himself increasingly as separate from the world, standing in opposition to it, as an I Seriousness and feelings of loneliness begin to stir in the child.[9] Perhaps he feels misunderstood by his surroundings, tends towards taking offence or dramatizes, and begins doubting familiar things by questioning the most natural things. It can happen that the child suddenly has the impression that his mother and father are not his real parents, but that he was exchanged at birth.

Almost every child goes through a crisis of loneliness. Often children experience insecurity in their social relationships, for example, not having a friend in their class or being cast out of their neighbourhood gangs etc. Physical weaknesses also occur like dizziness, a pounding heart or breathing difficulties. During this time the child needs lots of understanding and love from his surroundings to survive this phase without damage.[10]

Between the ninth and the twelfth years the child settles into his bone dynamic through his breathing process and through this experiences a certain objectivity of the will, which is organized into the world. While the child increasingly feels at home in his limbs, he experiences a new security on an unconscious level through growing world experience based on conceptual thinking. The child learns a new form of thinking, but does not yet master it.

Hans Müller-Wiedemann describes it as follows:

> 'The eleven-year-old seems to be ruled by its
> muscle system, which has -lost its early child-
> hood relationship to the blood organism and has
> emancipated itself without having reached its goal
> [...] Everything the child does or says appears to
> be wrong, whatever it takes into its hands breaks.
> It is full of wishes and desires but also sad when
> it is unpopular. — Sudden anger and unconcen-
> trated feelings are at the forefront of its moods. It
> does not do anything it is supposed to do, gives
> unsuited answers but can, much to the surprise of
> its mother, swear brilliantly. Its repertory of swear
> words is large. Its characteristics are: impulsiveness,
> quick reactions, directness and negativity. A turbu-
> lent age!'[11]

If we look at a twelve-year-old child, then a different personality reveals itself. He does not run or move in a carefree way
but rather sits and seems to have fallen into a heaviness to some

extent. He begins to stand more solidly on the earth. We also call this *earth maturity*. The relationship between parent and child starts to change. The critical time of the ninth to the twelfth year, with the ups and downs of incomprehensible feelings, moves into a new form of meeting. The children are looking for a more comradely relationship based on partnership. This has become possible through the newly-acquired ability to put themselves in the place of others, which reveals a first social responsibility. Now they have a different use of speech at every occasion ('awakening of the dialectic'). In family life this shows itself in numerous discussions, frequently paired with emerging provocation. The path towards the birth of a soul-body, into adolescence, is paved.

Example. *Fabian, just twelve years old, lives in a family with older and younger siblings. He has just left the previously described condition of lone-liness and insecurity in the family, and also school, behind him. He often felt left out in the class, as if he were in competition with the other boys. He was insecure and did not know what he wanted to be. Now his father describes how Fabian has suddenly started to lock the bathroom door, to create a private life. As part of this phenomenon he has also taken the door handle off his door so that nobody can just walk into his room. His mother is not allowed to point out how messy his school bag is or that he could use a shower. Fabian experiences this as getting-too-close, from which he has to distance himself brusquely. He enjoys the family conferences, and is the mem-ber who makes the clearest points and practises taking on a point of view. At the same time he does not spare criticism towards his parents.*

Puberty from fourteen to twenty-one years

In the previous chapter we saw how the seven year-old school child slowly begins to construct a thin emotional skin, which enables an ever increasing I experience. This emotional skin becomes denser and less permeable towards puberty, so that the teenager can now experience himself more strongly. This gives him the option and also the desire to be more self-contained. At the same time his emotions are roused. Suddenly the teenager feels that his life up until then with all the family habits, impressions, values and norms is something from the past, and he begins the search for the future. It is similar to what we have previously heard for the three year old: after a time of many impressions there follows a phase of expression, which has something to do with disassociation. This makes a teenager seem as if he has a sign hanging around his neck saying: closed for construction! Much of what he learnt during childhood is overthrown. 'In the soul of the growing child something like an inner spring clean occurs, and a lot of things are thrown out. Even if this spring clean is not expressed by difficult behaviour or a resistant attitude much can still be happening internally. The struggle for the future can be fought in a variety of different ways.'[12]

Every child expresses puberty in a different way. Jeanne Meijs categorizes the different ways into three basic types of puberty:

- First type: intellectual puberty;
- Second type: emotional puberty;
- Third type: will or action puberty.

Naturally each child goes through puberty with all three emotional types, but usually one of them is particularly intense. For a better understanding the three types are briefly described here:

Intellectual puberty

In a certain sense intellectual puberty is the transition from pre-puberty — when the new ability to speak emerges — into adolescence. The urges of the awakening I arises as thoughts in the soul, which is searching for itself. Adolescents start to discover the world with their thoughts. These can have a philosophical, religious, political or also deeply personal content, leading to deep discussions usually amongst their peers but also with great intensity in the family. The adolescents want to be taken seriously in their thoughts and to see 'behind the facade' of their parents and teachers, so that they can perceive new truthfulness in their relationships.

Important questions can be, for example:

- Does God really exist?
- Why does war happen?
- Who is the other human being?
- Does my teacher live what he asserts?
- What is a true friend?

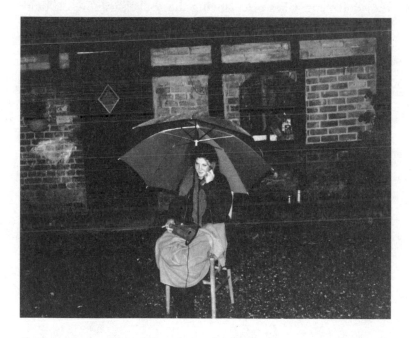

During puberty and the following years adolescents have a strong desire to distance themselves from the family and create their own area of life, which they should be granted.

Intellectual puberty, if followed too strongly, contains the danger of inner tension and hardening or circling thoughts.[13]

Emotional puberty

During emotional puberty the adolescent is caught between extremes of feelings, of sympathy and antipathy, one minute up and the next down. Here again we encounter the emotional skin. The antipathetic adolescent erects a protective barrier between itself and the outer world, in this way preparing himself for adulthood. During puberty the adolescent completely looses his child-like openness and learns instead to stand up for himself in the world. The I with its forces of the future lures this antipathy out of the youthful soul, which parents experience as bad moods and moroseness. A certain hardening around the soul of the adolescents takes place, giving the soul-skin more elasticity and making it more resilient.

The soul-skin of an adolescent experiencing sympathy is different. Sympathy has something to do with opening and widening, which often expresses itself in effusion, enthusiasm and passion. Teenagers worship idols, enjoy following fashion and lose themselves in music etc.

Loneliness, disappointment, illusion and disillusion belong to emotional puberty. For many adolescents their diary becomes an emotional companion, in which they tackle their feelings, often in the form of verse. In all emotions we can find the deep longing of the adolescent for himself. The emotional ups and downs cause the adolescent to become conscious of his own soul and the contents thereof, and leads to the realization that it is essential to become and remain a 'self.'[14]

Strongly-experienced emotional puberty can carry the danger of drug addiction, but also anorexia or depression.

Will puberty

This type of puberty is usually expressed by the strong desire to 'experiment' with life. The adolescent has the urge for direct experiences. Remember the first seven years, in which the child was a strong will person — this will can now be found again in a new form, enriched by personal life-experience. But the impulses are not penetrated by consciousness nor are the consequences of deeds overviewed, rather the adolescent just wants to do something, or to do nothing, as this can also be a form of will puberty. While one adolescent wants to transform each new idea into action, and demands direct freedom from his surroundings, the other falls into a bodily heaviness, cannot get out of bed anymore, refuses to go to school and discontinues everything with no interest in the consequences.

Externally teenagers often express their change of values by colouring their hair, having dreadlocks, consciously neglecting their appearance and getting their ears, nose and belly buttons pierced. Tattoos beautify the body and express current emotions.

Adolescents test relationships and seek sexual experiences. Sometimes they form lasting relationships, but more frequently experimentation reaches its peak. The adolescent searches for himself in meeting his peers.

This is also a time of separation from his parents, often the last one leading to independence and then to moving out of the parental home. Usually a new social awareness awakens in the adolescents, which often leads to a year of social work with elderly or disabled people. The sense of I in the form of a more liberated view of the other person has awakened. If there has not been too much conflict during puberty and the time thereafter, then a beautiful new phase of partnership begins between parents and 'child.'

4. It is Only With the Heart that One Can See Rightly

'Here is my secret. It is very simple: It is only
with the heart that one can see rightly; what is
essential is invisible to the eye.'

Antoine de Saint-Exupéry, *The Little Prince.*

The developmental phases of childhood have shown us how strongly childhood is subjected to processes of change and how much flexibility is demanded of parents if we want to do justice to each phase. We quickly loose sight of the child with her needs and opportunities, overload and overburden her with our opinion of how things should 'function,' and forget to keep a hold of life, of living things.

Antoine de Saint-Exupéry expresses this very aptly in the story of *The Little Prince,* by letting the fox say to the little prince on leaving: 'It is only with the heart that one can see rightly.'

This can also be interpreted in the following way: I only see the things in my surroundings, which leave an impression on my soul, which touch my heart. This is how the child relates to a flower, a stone, a screw, a snail, or to the vast starry sky and the moving clouds, to a human who looks at her, speaks to her and truly sees her.

How do I hear? When do I listen? Surely it is when something catches my interest, when a chord is struck in me and resounds. When does a child listen to what I want? Does she not listen to me when I have learnt to get involved with her instrument, when I am interested in the sound of her chords? If these are not tuned properly at the moment, so that the tones are discordant, there is no point in playing them loudly and firmly, rather I have to learn how to tune someone else's instrument. But I can also question the tones of my own instrument and what it needs to sound clearly and unambiguously.

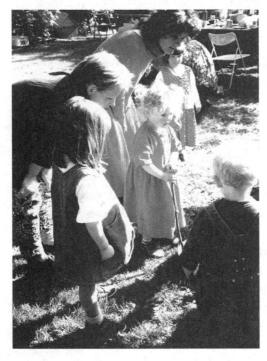

Children listen to us when we awaken their interest, when we play the strings of their soul instrument and make them resound.

Exercise A

Stock-taking

- Which of my sentences do I actually stand behind?
- What do I think of them? What do I really feel? How do I act?
- Which sentences are superfluous residues from my own upbringing?
- How often do I say things that I was hurt by when my parents said them to me?
- How much of what I say or do is actually out of loyalty towards my partner?

Exercise B

This exercise helps you to relate to the audible world:

- Listen consciously to the sounds and tones of day-to-day life.
- Take in the sounds of animals and listen to the expression of the soul that lies in them.
- Listen to the human voices in your surroundings, what do they express? How does the speech rhythm and sound affect you?

Fine tuning the instrument of the soul

Many receptive and observational capacities are needed to be able to manage family life with its different areas of work, or to work as a nanny or educator. It is only too easy for the language of the heart to get lost, which always has to do with attentiveness, patience, tolerance and acceptance towards the stranger.

Where do we get the inspiration from to preserve these qualities in education or in social relationships? Language helps us further with the term 'presence of mind,' as it signifies bringing a moment of thought into a present situation otherwise dominated by emotional entanglement. Presence of mind in the widest sense means: the ability to be conscious, or the I-force as a perceptive organ for the soul.

All too quickly our soul seems like an unrehearsed orchestra without a conductor. Our thoughts, feelings and actions often roam through it without purposeful guidance through the I, the conductor within us.

Rudolf Steiner recommends a variety of exercises especially for schooling the soul forces, which can be found in Chapter 12. It can be very effective to devote oneself to a small, self-chosen task for at least five minutes a day. This can be a concentration or observational exercise challenging one's consciously engaged will or a determined quality of thinking: for example, positive thinking or the decision to remain impartial in certain situations. This kind of self-discipline strengthens the life-forces, emotions and the I of the human being, which then shows its effect on upbringing.

One can become conscious of one's personal weaknesses and strengths, and what one needs at that moment, by asking the question to what extent one feels at home at the moment in one's body, soul and I-forces. A state of tiredness and exhaustion shows my life-forces are weakened, which usually means I also feel emotionally imbalanced and have little sense for myself. In this situation it might be necessary for me to do something for myself, seemingly egotistically, as the short freedom experienced thereby often leads surprisingly to a better perception of the other people in my life. If my children and partner are involved in this process, then I am also creating the basis for developing understanding.

If we look back to Chapter 2 using this point of view, to Susan and her sons (p. 16), then perhaps we can better understand her reactions. But Susan's sons were not able to comprehend her behaviour. They probably could have done so if Susan had talked about her exhaustion, asked for a break and then arranged to meet up for a conversation. So 'Listen to what I say' takes on the sense of 'Say what is happening, so I can understand you!'

The same is true for the conflict I mentioned with my daughter (see p. 16–17). She felt wounded and subtly pushed away. How differently it would have sounded if I had said: 'This is my first free evening for a long time and I would really like to be alone. It has nothing to do with you. I would be glad if you could understand it.'

The situation is different for Josefa and little Antonella (see p. 15). Josefa tries to give her small daughter instructions on the side, which is actually too much for her. Antonella still needs direct speech and attention to be able to act. Added to this Antonella also notices Josefa's increasing tension and inner turmoil and reacts like a small seismograph. Antonella can only be happy again once Josefa pays direct attention to her, and manages to re-organize herself with a quiet internal dialogue.

'Listen to what I say' in the sense of 'What is speaking in me?' can then become an inner dialogue where I am listener and speaker at the same time. This sets the scene for listening with the heart.

I have had the most exciting conversations and conflicts with myself. 'Inner mother speaks to inner child.' How lovingly or how strictly do I treat myself? How does this affect my children and partner? Depending on the circumstances I react with rebellion, withdrawal or an open heart. Yes, and often enough I have to act in accordance with what I have attained through reasoning, depending how well I have learnt to work as the director of the different players on the internal stage.

The exercises described below help to open as many doors as possible which free the way from head to heart and nourish the moment of 'presence of mind.'

Looking into the heart of the child

Listen to your children and look at them:

- When do I see pain flicker in their eyes?
- When do they push out their chin in defence?
- When do they stiffen their back in anger and defiance?
- When are they under pressure and threaten to explode?
- When do their eyes become clear and their back soft?
- When are they happy and feel secure?
- When do they cry from natural and necessary frustration?
- When do they cry from sadness or fear?

5. Speak, and You Reveal Yourself

Understand the sense of speech,
And the world reveals
Itself as image.

Hear the soul of speech,
And the world opens
Itself as being.

Experience the spirit of speech,
And the world bestows
Power of wisdom.

Love speech itself
And it confers on you
Its own power.

So will I turn heart and ear
To spirit and soul
Of the Word;

And in the love of speech
I experience
My own self.

Rudolf Steiner[16]

Body language, soul language

Speech, beside touch, is the most direct connection between mother, father and child. Much lies hidden within it: a voice can sound soft or hard. Pronunciation can be indistinct or well articulated, the tone high pitched or deep. Our emotions are revealed through speech, our mood is shown by our voice. Perhaps a voice sounds broken, hoarse or loud and we hear insecurity, sadness, anger, decisiveness or happiness in it. A person's mood can be heard in its voice. We can perceive the human being by listening to its voice, as it is connected to the essence of a person in a unique way. Its carrier is our red, warm blood, which means we can lend an emotional content to our voice and express our I-force.[17] The iron in the blood, which gives it its red colour, is responsible for this phenomenon on a material level. People who have experienced iron deficiency can perhaps remember their lack of energy to do things and their weaker, feeble voice. Our voice, forming sounds and guided by breathing, reveals our inner fire and our I-presence in the blood and is also shown by our posture. Rudolf Steiner described the metamorphosis from physical gestures to voice modulations to actors and speech therapists in the following way:[18]

GESTURE	VOICE
1. effective, direct	Cutting
2. reflective	Full
3. questioning	Quivering
4. antipathetic	Hard
5. sympathetic	Soft
6. withdrawn	Short, sharp

We can sense how our emotions are expressed in our voice through tone (pitch and modulation). The voice receives a cutting, guided character if I want to express my will. If, however, I am still contemplating what to say while speaking, my voice has a deliberate, fuller sound which shows that I am still occupied with myself, with my thoughts, rather than engaged with the other person. An uncertain, quivering voice shows I am asking a question. When I reject something my voice sounds hard, but becomes soft when I feel sympathetic towards someone or something. If I retreat inwardly and emotionally, then my voice also sounds as if it is retreating. Our voice makes audible what gestures show in space, and we can observe in what way, and with which emotion, the soul is connecting to the world. This information invites you to pay attention to your own voice to receive an idea of your personal emotional demeanour.

In this way we can discover something about the sound of speech. This fact alone has an effect on the listener, and is meaningful for bringing up children. Children are brought up on the one hand by our emotional example, but equally important is our speech which affects children right into their physical development (see Chapters 3 and 5 about the development of the child).

Nowadays, one can already notice a deformation of the child's speech organs due to a lack of example in their surroundings. Too little is spoken, sung or read out loud in the family and instead technical, soul-less voices from television and audiotapes have taken over.

Up to now we have looked at audible speech, which is usually supported by the 'speaking body.' But we also use non-verbal speech, expressing attitudes without words: a wish, an accusation, joy or disappointment. Often non-verbal gestures like facial expression, sighing, laughing and clicking tongues play a large part in upbringing, as in the example of Family D:

Family D is sitting at the supper table; the parents and their three children are conversing together animatedly. While the fourteen-year-old son is talking about his experiences at school his mother repeatedly raises her eyebrows. Eventually the son asks her: 'What's wrong?' even though Mrs D has not said anything. When she answers: 'Nothing, go on, I'm interested in everything you're saying,' her son appears slightly confused and uncertain.

A short while later Mrs D mentions she would like to go to the cinema and asks her husband whether he would like to join her. Mr D wrinkles his forehead and says: 'All right, if you want me to!'

Mrs D counters: 'You obviously don't want to go!'

Mr D: 'No, I didn't say that!'

Mrs D: 'But it showed in your face.'

Mr D: 'You need to believe what I said.'

Mrs D with an irritated undertone: 'Well, are you coming or not?'

The members of Family D are not quite sure who means what, as so many covert messages are sent.

This example shows how non-verbal statements can confuse and contribute towards conflict. If my words express one message and simultaneously my body language transmits a different message, then I am split between my deliberate and unconscious statements. Non-verbal statements are usually more truthful and less distorted by hopes and desires or by what people think they should be saying. Usually non-verbal statements convey what I really mean, while spoken words express what I imagine or intend to do. Sometimes non-verbal statements do not contradict the spoken words, but add important information to them.

It is helpful to pay more attention to non-verbal messages. Once they have been consciously grasped they can strengthen communication and help us find solutions for the real problems within a partnership. Particularly children are very sensitive and quickly pick up and internalize covert messages, and then, at some point, they begin to influence the child's behaviour. Observing our own non-verbal gestures can help us to understand our emotions and reveal reasons for existing conflicts.

Exercises

For partners and parental groups

- Sit down opposite a partner and look at one another. Say things to your partner that you deliberately cancel out through a non-verbal gesture. Invalidate the meaning of what you said by your movements, facial expressions, the tone of your voice, laughing, etc. Observe each other while doing so, pay attention to what you and your partner do to cancel out the spoken message. Discuss the results together.
- Sit opposite a partner: one of you mirrors the language and the facial expression of the other. The one says anything whatsoever; the other immediately repeats what has been said

as quickly and accurately as possible, using the same volume, inflection, facial expressions and head movements. Try to copy the expression of your partner exactly and perceive how he transmits his message. — Change roles and discuss your experiences with each other.

The meaning of the voice for educating hearing

Each newborn child has the deep longing to settle into earthly conditions. Month after month, year after year she increasingly inhabits her body (incarnation), so as to be able to take hold of life's tasks. We have heard how important it is that as parents we accompany our children in their development, and that speech, beside touch, is the most direct connection between mother, father and child. We can hear the soul's mood in the voice and recognize the individual person by their voice. Each one of us has a unique emotional tone of voice, which reveals the 'primal colouring of our self' and creates a 'space' where our human soul inhabits our body.

Some voices resound out of the chest area, others more out of the head; the latter always sounds high, often metallic, and can seem grating and annoying if over-emphasized, sometimes producing a hectic atmosphere. By contrast, a voice sounding from the chest area is warm and enveloping, darker, but perhaps also lethargic and monotonous. Other examples of pitches are a nasal or tight voice. All these voice images show how much the voice can be connected in one-sidedness to the body.

We have also seen how our emotions are revealed through our voice's tone, inflection and modulation, and through its gesture. With our characteristic tenor we affect the breathing, and with that the mood of the other person, our child. At the same we also try to hear how our child is feeling, pick up her mood, by the sound of her voice. One can experience this clearly in the relationship between parents and newborns. In particular the mother can hear whether her child is contented or not by the sound of its voice. Children are also quick to pick up what people in their surrounding are feeling, sometimes their voice sounds impatient or happy, at other times calm or loving.

I think it has become clear what a great social responsibility we have in relation to our own voice and speech. I would briefly like to mention that speech plays an important part in the child's development, as through speech the child shapes her inner organs. In particular, the brain, which is still quite 'shapeless' after birth, can be structured through well-formed speech. This then leads to the development of a clear and ordered consciousness.

As mentioned at the start of this book more and more parents feel unsure about bringing up their children, which is naturally also revealed by their voice. Taking the above information into account we can sense what a fundamental effect this insecurity has on the child's development. Often the tone of voice is 'heady,' too thin and high and unconsciously rises upwards towards the end of a sentence. This in turn signals to the chil-

Often we do not consider how important language is for the child – not only for speech development, but also for its physical development.

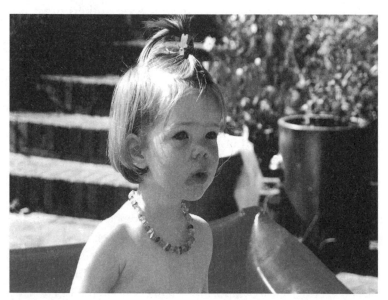

dren that the parents are asking them a question or do not know themselves how they should relate to a particular situation.

The child's reaction to this way of speaking is that she neither feels adequately spoken to, nor touched inside by what she has heard.

The very young child needs speech and inflection to incarnate. Birth completes her downward path from heaven to earth after which she then wants to assimilate to the world. She does not want to be 'drawn out' again by the questioning attitude and insecurity of her parents. But the abovementioned tone of voice leads to this tendency.

A full and clear voice which is guided from a high to a low pitch reaches the child right in her physical organism, while a high-pitched, questioning voice remains 'outside' and easily creates an irritable mood. Children require clarity and sureness in our speech and accompanying gestures, as it helps them to develop feelings of support and security. Each theatrical speech with a moral or intellectual undertone goes against this feeling, as it creates insecurity and nervousness. This is the case for children before they reach school age.

The child calls out to us: 'Speak to me so I can hear you!'

Exercises for partner or parent's groups[19]

Identifying with your voice

Decide who should be A and who B. Close your eyes if it helps you to concentrate and centre yourself. Let A listen to his own voice as he speaks and describe what it conveys as if he himself were this voice. For example: 'I am my voice. I am soft and slow swaying a little up and down. I sound a bit reproachful, as if I want to ask for something.'

Listen to your voice exactly and pay attention to what you can still discover in it.

During this time B should be quiet and carefully listen to the voice of his partner. Pay exact attention to the characteristics of the voice, observe all feelings, impressions or images which arise within you while listening. Continue this for several minutes …

Now exchange roles. A listens to B, B identifies with his voice and describes it for several minutes.

Open your eyes and tell your partner what you have noticed while listening to his voice, also mention the emerging images. Both of you should attempt to describe the characteristic of the sounds and also what these sounds and pauses mean to you!

Dialogue between parent and child

Let A be father or mother, B the child. Speak to each other as if you were these roles. Say what you like but pay close attention to what you say, what your pitch expresses, how you feel and how you interact with your partner. Continue this for several minutes.

Now exchange roles, B is father or mother, A is the child. Again converse for several minutes and observe what happens between you.

Sit still and think about what you have experienced. Clarify what kind of parent you are and what kind of child. As a parent are you cold, authoritarian, clever, loving, suggestive, etc.? And as a child: Are you whiny, obliging, rebellious, do you take on an apologetic attitude etc.?

Try to clarify the atmosphere and the details of this role-play between parent and child. How did you experience your partner in his role as a parent or a child? Which positive and negative structures and qualities could you observe in each other etc.?

Speech exercises which train articulation and guide will-power into speech:

Tongue twisters

1 Peter Piper picked a peck of pickled peppers.
   A peck of pickled peppers Peter Piper picked.
   If Peter Piper picked a peck of pickled peppers,
   Where's the peck of pickled peppers Peter Piper picked?

2 She sells seashells on the sea shore.
   The shells she sells are seashells, I'm sure.

3   There's no need to light a night–light
    On a light night like tonight
    For a night–light's a slight light
    On a light night like tonight.

4   Betty bought a bit of butter.
    But, she said, this butter's bitter.
    If I put it in my batter, it will make my batter bitter.
    So she bought a bit of butter, better than her bitter butter,
    And she put it in her batter, and her batter was not bitter.
    So 'twas better Betty bought a bit of better butter.

5   Swan swam over the sea
    Swim, swan, swim!
    Swan swam back again
    Well swum, swan!

6   Round and round the rugged rocks the ragged rascal ran.

7   A flee and a fly in a flue
    Were imprisoned, so what could they do?
    Said the fly let us flee,
    Said the flee let us fly,
    So they flew through the flaw in the flue.

Say these tongue twisters faster and faster without mistakes. Have fun!

6. Speaking, Listening and Understanding

The following conversation is typical at the breakfast table of a couple presumably married for decades.

The dialogue starts with the words: 'Berta, the egg is hard!'

Her laconic answer is: 'I heard you!'

He goes on: 'How long was the egg boiled?'

She answers; 'Too many eggs are not healthy at all!'

When he insists on knowing for how long this particular egg has been boiled she answers: 'You always want to have it cooked for four and half minutes.'

This conversation continues in this manner for a while, until he finally counters with the question: 'Then why is my breakfast egg too hard sometimes and too soft at other times?'

'I don't know ... I'm not a hen!'

During the further discussion about the exact cooking time she finally comes up with her 'having a feeling for it' as a housewife.

He answers: 'But it is hard ... perhaps something is wrong with your feeling ...'

'Something is wrong with my feeling? I stand in the kitchen all day, do the washing, tidy up your things, tidy the house, struggle with the children and you say something is wrong with my feeling?'

'All I asked for was a soft egg ... I don't care how long it has been boiled!'

'Oh, you don't care if I spend four and a half minutes working in the kitchen!'

In the further course of the discussion he is not given the chance to talk again, apart from single protests. Eventually her annoyance ends with the exclamation: 'My god, men are so primitive.' And she breaks off the conversation.

He ends the conflict with an inner dialogue: 'I'm going to kill her …
tomorrow I'm going to kill her.'[20]

This example shows the classic development of a misunder-
standing, the kind we possibly all know, if more moderately.
Conversations like this can quickly develop particularly between
family members or friends. Strengths, weaknesses and touchi-
ness of the other members are all too well known, as are their
assumed reactions to what is going to be said. Some families use
this kind of communication without even realizing how much
relationships suffer from it. Speaking, listening and understanding are deeds which cannot be left to themselves. Parents and
partners need to increasingly take on the responsibility for them
and remain conscious of them. To help achieve this the following
section deals with the content and different levels of the spoken
words. Communication always takes place between two people,
the one sends a message and the other receives it. Sometimes
we can be quite surprised by the message the other has received.
Often conversations lead to misunderstandings and well-meant
pedagogical discipline ends in opposition, neither of which has
anything in common with the actual matter of concern.

Sending four messages

When I stand in the hallway in the morning and shout through
the house with an admonitory tone of voice that it is already
7.30AM — by which I actually mean that the children should
hurry up so as not to be late for school — then it should not
surprise me if I am hit by waves of irritation from all sides.
Alternatively it is also possible that my son shouts: 'Yes, I know,
thanks.'

A single message, sent to different people, can be heard and
processed in completely different ways. As a result I would like
to clarify the 'anatomy' of messages, using a diagram according
to Friedemann Schulz von Thun.[21]

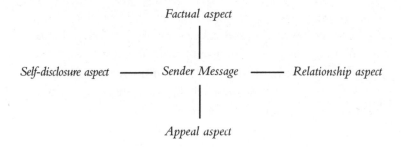

First we have the sender, the person who wants to communicate something. Then we have the message, which is what the sender would like to say. My message was: 'It is 7.30AM.' I, as the sender, can be sending out different statements with this message. These can be organized into the following aspects:

1. The factual aspect
This level conveys the specific information; the factual message is of primary importance. In our example the clock shows the time, 7.30AM.

2. The self-disclosure aspect
In this case I disclose something about myself as well as the factual information. In our example: I have an eye on the time, am worried and already slightly irritated as the children will probably be late if they do not hurry up. Friedemann Schulz von Thun calls this compulsory self-portrayal, or also involuntary self-exposure.[22] This kind of message often leads to communication problems between people and causes complicated transactions, which we will look at in more detail later.

3. The relationship aspect
A message also reveals my relationship to the listener, what I think of him. This is often conveyed by the tone of voice, body language and gestures (see also Chapter 5). The listener can feel badly treated by these signals. In our example this might mean that my children feel criticized or that I am deciding things for them, or that I do not trust them to pay attention to the time themselves.

4.The appeal aspect

This aspect of the message reveals an underlying demand and a covert desire to make the other person do something. The message tries to motivate the receiver to do or not do certain things, but can also relate to thoughts or feelings. In the above example the appeal to the children might be:

- Try harder;
- Hurry up;
- Don't dawdle;
- Don't do anything unnecessary.
- Don't clean your teeth etc.

Even if appeal and relationship aspects are closely related, they should be differentiated, as the same appeal can have different relationship messages. How the listener receives the message does not only depend on the message, but also on his mood.

Thus my son reacts calmly and factually, and in contrast to his sister he answers: 'Yes, I know, thanks:'

Receiving with four ears

The following section explains these four different message aspects from the point of view of the receiver. Depending which aspect of the message the listener listens to predominantly, he will hear a different message. Actually he is not listening with two ears, but with four:

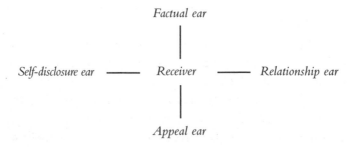

Factual ear

Self-disclosure ear ——— *Receiver* ——— *Relationship ear*

Appeal ear

1. The factual ear

Our example (see p. 54) shows that my son was listening mainly to my covert demand with his factual ear. Correspondingly he answered on a 'factual' level. Perhaps he was in a happy mood so that he did not take my covert message personally.

The inner question asked with the factual ear is: how are the facts to be understood?

2. The relationship ear

My son would have probably reacted differently if he had been listening with his relationship ear. He might have felt personally attacked and become aggressive.

Some children have a particularly well-developed relationship ear. They immediately relate the message to themselves, easily feel attacked or insulted, or get the impression they are being laughed at. This makes them react defensively (see also Chapter 9, the section 'Aggression as a warning sign').

On this level the receiver asks the question: What does the sender think of me? Who does he think I am and how do I feel treated?

3. The self-disclosure ear

Unlike the above case, the self-disclosure ear reveals nothing about the receiver. Instead, the receiver gets a close look at the sender in the sense of: So that is who you are! My son perhaps thought quietly: My goodness, mother has had too little sleep again — with which he protected himself against the covert attack. Children are only able to do this after they are about seven years old, until then they hear unclear messages solely with their relationship ear.

Messages with this aspect are processed with the question: What does this message say about you?

4. The appeal ear

The messages received by the appeal ear are examined in relationship to their appeal character. What does mother or father expect of me? What should I think, feel or do? A receiver with 'big appeal ears' is usually less centred in themselves and often tries to be obedient and do everything correctly.

For this theory to become practice take a look at yourself with regard to your four ears and four senders. You will probably have many questions; this shows you are on the right path.[23]

For a deeper and broader understanding of the phenomenon of the different sending and receiving modes I would like to look at the transaction analysis model. It has stood me in good stead both in my personal life and in my work. Personally, I think Schulz von Thun's communication theory can be linked up well with the transaction analysis, as he also

Was the sent message received in the right way?

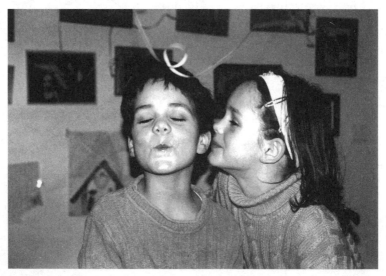

bases his explanations on different inner experiences which have an effect on social life. He calls them:

• The network of systematic connections around me; and
• Emotional cooperation and conflict within myself.

In the following chapters I would like to show you these relationships and their deeper levels.

7. Transaction Analysis and Bringing up Children

Parents, children and adults in one person

In the last chapter we discussed the different informational messages sent or received and noticed that we react differently depending on mood and childhood experiences. It can also be a great help to find out consciously which 'role' we use when speaking. This chapter aims to introduce you to your 'inner child,' the 'inner parents' and the adult in yourself.

Eric Berne, the founder of transaction analysis, observed during his psychosomatic counselling that within short periods of time people noticeably altered their behaviour. Their voices, attitude and facial expression changed and with that their feelings and opinions.

He calls these changing conditions, which we can observe in ourselves, Ego States or personality parts. These are created in early childhood and are carried within us throughout our lives. The neurobiologist, Gerald Hüther, speaks of neural connections in the brain, which are responsible for the basic forms of individually conditioned thoughts, feelings and actions.[24]

Berne describes how people often underline their words with gestures when talking about themselves, for example, they furrow their brow as if parents are talking critically to a child, or they say something mediating, comforting. In this state they are acting out of their Parent Ego State (P).

The Parent Ego State

Each one of us is familiar with leading inner dialogues, talking to oneself. We can act in two different ways with our Parent: in a caring, supporting way and a correcting, controlling and criticizing way. The nurturing Parent helps, comforts, and looks after others or itself, like loving adults for a child. The critical Parent, which we unfortunately often embody, can have a harsh effect with threatening, forbidding and fear-provoking actions, bursts of feeling and gestures. The Parent also keeps track of the necessary rules, demands and prohibitions as well as attaining survival and life-mastering skills. Our Parent Ego State acts according to our ideas and values, norms and rules and is often also prejudiced. It is our learned concept of life.

Physical and verbal clues which reveal that we are acting from our Parent Ego State are: knitted eyebrows, clicking tongue, furrowed brow, sighing, pointed lips, head patting, pointed forefinger, wringing one's hands, horrified lifting of eyes, arms folded in front of chest.

The following expressions are also uttered from the Parent Ego State:

'I'll make sure that this stops immediately ...'
'I can't stand it when ...'
'You always have to remember that ...'
'You must never forget, that ...'
'How often have I told you ...'
'If I were you ...'

Words that point towards prejudices can be:
— stupid, outrageous, lazy, ridiculous, messy, disgusting etc.
— 'poor thing,' 'little child,' 'very clever,' 'again,' 'idiot,' 'what now?'

Suggestion
Get to know your parent. Pay attention to the kind of non-verbal messages you send to your family. How do the others react to it? Which words constitute your vocabulary when you speak to your children or partner? Which inner dialogue do you lead with your own inner child?

The Adult Ego State

A person who thinks, explains, reports or informs himself is acting out of a different Ego State. He speaks factually and calmly and has an upright stance when speaking; his voice is relatively monotonous. Berne calls this the *Adult* Ego State *(A)*. Our Adult helps us to make decisions and gain clarity in situations. We can test our actions using the Adult Ego State and have better control over our emotions. We can observe that even unpleasant feelings are very important and helpful if we use our Adult to fathom them, and can then act to change our situation. I ask questions and receive information with my Adult.

Acting out of our Adult Ego State is expressed in the following way: our face shows interest, is open and facing towards our partner. When listening, movements like nodding or signs of agreement (mmh) are noticeable.

Speech clues are words or phrases like:

— why, how much, what, who, how;
— I think, I believe, I mean;
— Possibly, probably, etc.

Suggestion

How do you react to conflicts? Do you become emotional very quickly, or do you start an inner dialogue using your thoughts?

Do you ask questions about the circumstances or do you intervene immediately?

The Child Ego State

A further ego state is revealed by behaviours similar to those of a child. We are in this state when we are happy, laughing, crying or also angry, rebellious, or unwilling to do something just because it is demanded of us. In this state we can be creative, inconsiderate, sympathetic and have fun. Berne calls this the *Child Ego State (C)*. This Child is the source of our energy if it can flow freely.

Eric Berne organizes the Child Ego States into three categories: a free, an adapted and a rebellious Child. The adapted part is dependant on authority, follows rules, demands, prohibitions and norms, for example: 'One does not speak with a full mouth!' or 'children should listen.'

The rebellious Child Ego State needs to revolt or go against something.

In the Child the person experiences an inner image of his life's concept. He feels basic emotions like anger, love, sadness, happiness, envy, disgust and hatred. Because of this we say an emotional person has been taken over by his Child.

The Child reveals creativity, curiosity, thirst for knowledge, pleasure in touch. He stores beautiful and negative memories.

Physical clues pointing towards the Child Ego State are, for example: tears, trembling lips, sudden temper tantrums, a high, whiny voice, shrugging shoulders, laughing, making faces, pleading, biting nails, lowered eyes etc.

Verbal clues are phrases like:
'I want …,' 'I wish …,' 'I don't know …,' 'I am now going to do …,' large, larger, largest … superlatives!

Suggestion
Get to know your Child and think about what percentage of the different Ego States you are. Which Child Ego State are you the most or the least?

Eric Berne has arranged these Ego States within each person into this diagram (see opposite page).

These ego states can also be described as personality parts. We do not have immediate access to them all from birth, they develop during the course of childhood.

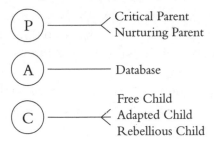

In the following section I refer to Eric Berne's later colleagues. They related transaction analysis to childhood and adolescence. Even if there are temporal differences in this description of the child's development to the anthroposophical study of the human being, I think these proposals are both exciting and helpful for upbringing and creating relationships.[25]

The development of personality parts

Up until six months of age

A newborn child only has one of the ego states mentioned above to relate to its parents. This state is called 'the Child in the child,' the 'biological child' or the 'free child.'[26] From birth up until about six months the baby almost solely reacts with anything that will get attention. He cries when he is hungry, thirsty or tired. He does not have any feeling for time and does not know how long it will take for somebody to attend to him. The child starts broadening this ego state from day one through experiences.

During this developmental phase it needs parents using all three ego states. The nurturing Parent lovingly gives it food and protection. Our Adult Ego State gathers information about the correct way to handle the child, who to entrust it to, how to feed it, which paediatrician to choose etc. Our own inner child helps us to empathize with the feelings and needs of the baby. We can ask ourselves what would make us content if we were in the baby's position (see the exercise on p. 77).

This early dependant relationship can also be called symbiosis. It protects the life of the child. All the experiences of this first age are 'stored' in the 'free child' as memories, which give feelings of trust and security, but can also be a first basis for insecurity and lack of trust.

Example: *Frederick has just learnt to walk. He walks through the house on unsteady legs but his desire to discover has been awakened. He pulls himself up everywhere and already tries to reach the table by pulling the things towards him with the tablecloth. He wants to copy his mother. Although she is proud of Frederick's progress, her critical Parent admonishes him all the time: 'Watch out! Don't drop that! No, don't touch that!' Frederick feels uncertain. Sometimes his mother is even quite loud, and then he gets a fright, falls down onto his bottom and gazes introspectively.*

The ego state of a baby can be shown systematically in the following way: the 'child-I in the child' is the only ego state developed.

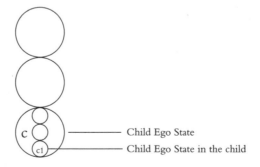

From six to eighteen months

Between six and eighteen months the Child Ego State is extended by a further personality part, the 'Adult in the Child.' This has nothing to do with the later developing Adult (see p.63). This 'Adult in the Child' is sometimes called the 'little crafty thing,' with which the child listens to the mood of the surrounding.[27] This is the basis of our intuition or a pre-conscious ability to 'know' what is happening.

The child is now increasingly able to remember things and have elementary experiences of the senses and movement, and once it has learnt to stand up then speech and thinking soon develop.

The child still needs a symbiotic relationship to parents who use all three ego states. With our Parent and Adult we give our children the space to discover their surroundings. We allow them to follow their desire for experiencing the world. A home where children continuously come up against limits — where there are things they are not allowed to touch, they are not allowed to get dirty or not allowed to eat by themselves in case they make a mess — holds back the free inner child and teaches him to rebel already during this early age. In contrast the child feels nurtured if his parents can sense what the child needs at any given time using their Child Ego State.

The nurturing Parent Ego State gives the child approval and encourages him to discover his surroundings. Fearful and over-protective parents tend to continuously accompany their children verbally, which blocks their independent development. 'Watch out! Don't fall down there! Don't go so far away!' These demands come from a critical Parent Ego State and stop children making their own experiences.

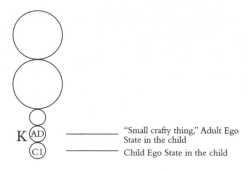

K (AD) ————— "Small crafty thing," Adult Ego State in the child
(C1) ————— Child Ego State in the child

From eighteen to thirty-six months

Between eighteen months and three years the child's sppech and thinking abilities increase and improve. First he learns to name the outer world: dog, table, mug, doll, milk etc. He recognizes objects and gives them the correct term. This is the start of a verbal standing against the outside world; before this the child still felt completely connected to the world. Learning to speak starts a process of disassociation of the self from the world as a whole; this process culminates at about two and a half with the obstinate stage. By the time the child has reached this stage he has learnt, through his developing speech, to think in three great steps: naming the things in his surroundings has led to the realization that they are distinctive objects. Through thinking and speaking he experiences the relationship between objects: drink milk, dog barks, doll sleeping etc. and learns to comprehend these relationships. This gives the child an elementary sense of time. The feeling for today, tomorrow, yesterday awakens and the child learns to recognize simple, later also complicated, relationships which are connected to actions.

A sense of his own being arises in the child during this phase of thinking. The own I awakens! When the child experiences his I he begins to remember things consciously. Now the child longs for more independence and autonomy. Everything captures his interest and leads to questions. The child starts asking 'why' at every turn. Rüdiger Rogoll attributes a largely functional, developing Adult Ego State to the child.[28] The child even questions familiar things and experiments with his wishes and his new feeling for himself and the world. 'No, I don't want to' becomes his favourite sentence.[29] The child begins to further separate from his parents. Using the Adult Ego State as much as possible to meet the child, and not the rebellious Child or the critical Parent, helps to reduce the stress which parents are subjected to during this time.

> 'Their Adult helps them think about which rules
> and demands they want to implement, whether
> their actions are sensible, whether their child is
> able to make decisions, for example when eat-
> ing [...] It is important that parents concentrate
> solely on essential rules to protect the child [...].
> Parents can sense with their C (Child) if the
> child is scared alone in the dark, and then leave
> the door open or a lamp on. Many problems can
> be mastered with humour using the inner child.
> Children need parents who are 'happy to play'
> [...]. The child needs protection, patience and
> encouragement from the nurturing Parent to be
> able to cope with its wavering feelings, its need to
> separate from its parents, its wanting-to-be-small-
> again.'[30]

When children of this age are gripped by obstinacy, confronting them with the critical Parent Ego State can sometimes help them regain their composure.

Example: *Lucas is two and a half years old. He is very strong and has started saying 'no' to everything. If he senses resistance he becomes even more unyielding. Today he wants to play outside.*
  Lucas: 'I want to go outside!'
  Mother: 'Yes, come here, I'll put your coat on.'
  Lucas: 'I want to go out without my coat!'

Mother: 'No, it's too cold:'
Lucas: 'But I don't want to go out with my coat!'
Mother: 'No …'

The conversation goes back and forth in this manner for a few minutes. Arguments, tricks, games, nothing works. Lucas throws himself to the ground and screams, hits his head against the floor and screams even louder. The mother starts shouting: 'Stop crying now, I can't understand you when you're like this and I can't help you either!' She holds him tight and looks at him with a strict gaze. Lucas manages to compose himself, he still cries a bit, but only mildly.

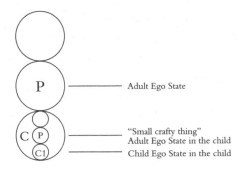

From three to six years

The period of obstinacy strengthens the I of the child during his fourth year and lets him become an increasingly expressive being. The child widens his sphere of action more and more and tries to understand relationships with his Adult Ego State.

Rüdiger Rogoll believes that the child now starts developing an early 'Parent Ego State in the child,' P1.[31] The child does this by emulating the restraining and caring behaviour of his parents, which creates the space and the example for his own happiness and joyful playing. His power of imagination is now fully developed. This in turn strengthens the joy and creativity which nurtures the child's play and social behaviour. He discovers rules, tests their strength and increasingly finds out what other people expect of him. The child starts thinking about other people and trying out parental behaviour, whether it be educating the dog or lovingly looking after, or admonishing, a younger sibling.

One can see touching scenes when one watches children playing with their doll or teddy bear, as this is where the early Parent Ego State in the child emerges. Often the birth of a younger sibling makes the still young child use his Adult and Parent Ego States at the same time as he also uses his rebellious and adapted Child Ego State.

An example from my surgery: a mother with two children aged four and one takes up educational counselling because she is troubled by the change in her four-year-old daughter. The child has become quieter and is always careful to help her mother. The latter is in a state of extreme exhaustion and often feels more like a child. She has the impression that her daughter wants to manage the housework like a little adult mother and is actually completely out of her depths. Once the mother can take over her role as the adult again, if necessary with outside help, then the daughter can perhaps start playing again as well as being a little helper.

During this age group the parents still need to be there for their children using all three Ego States, but gradually other people start to influence the child as well, for example nursery teachers, neighbours and playmates and their parents.

Parents should take their child seriously and be willing to compromise. This shows the child how to solve problems by thinking them through. He or she needs: 'protection, caring, and corrections from the Parent Ego State. Parents set limits using their critical Parent, sometimes also taking a standing against others.'[32] If, for example, a grandparent says to her crying grandson: 'But boys don't cry!' then the parent has to think about whether it is necessary to correct this statement to avoid negative associations in the child.

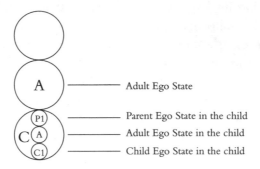

Adult Ego State

Parent Ego State in the child
Adult Ego State in the child
Child Ego State in the child

From six to twelve years

As we have already seen in Chapter 3, the child increasingly separates from its family during this phase, and interacts more with friends and peers. He experiences how other families have different values and standards, and that the rules and methods of the teachers at school can be different from those in the parental home. The child questions existing rules and prohibitions, makes up his own rules and opposes familiar habits. Children not only test their parents, but also their teachers and neighbours, playing tricks on them or disregarding their limits.

The child now starts developing its Parent Ego State.

> 'The Parent Ego State is created, modified and augmented over the years by experiences made with the environment and particularly with people of authority and people who are important to us. The more messages we can store which are supportive and strengthen self-confidence, the more effective is the protection that the Parent can afford us. Even critical messages can help us to find our way.'[33]

But if critical messages predominate in upbringing then children cannot develop sufficient self-confidence, and they get the feeling that they are 'not normal,' while they think others are 'normal.' If, during this age, the parents manage not to rigidly insist on their values and ideas, but learn to value the growing Adult and the creative free Child in their children, then they lay the foundations for a constructive Parent Ego State.

The development of the child's personality also necessitates parental growth. If, for example, the ten-year-old son wants to go to bed later than his younger sister, then this request can become an impulse to discuss such questions together with all the members of the family in a 'family conference' (see also Chapter 11). Parents develop simultaneously with their children when they take time for their children and pay attention to the changing needs of different ages.

Parents still need to make their three ego states available to their child between the ages of six and twelve, but in an adapted way. As partners of their children parents meet them with their Adult Ego State and help them to clarify facts, which makes them into an example for critical and constructive thinking. Using their Adult they can question family agreements. They can show their child the relationship between cause and effect to teach him the importance of assuming responsibility, and offer him a personal point of view.

You do not need to empathize with the child with your own Child anymore, as you can now ask him how he is feeling. But you can do the child a great favour by playing games with him, going swimming, sailing or skating. The element of joy and liveliness stems from the energy of the Child Ego State.

The child still needs the Parent Ego State of his parents and other adults for protection and to find his way in life. The certainty that he is allowed to distance himself from home, but is also welcome when he comes back again, strengthens his self-confidence. Instead of criticizing the children when they are fighting with others, we can help with questions like: 'If you were Catherine, how would you feel?' This teaches the child to use his own different personality parts.

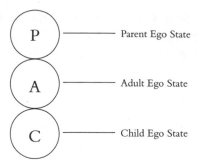

From thirteen to nineteen years

By this time adolescents have developed all three ego states and only need to expand and augment them. Particularly during puberty this means they need the space to practise them.

The adolescent takes over more and more responsibility, enabling him to learn to solve problems both with regard to himself and others. We have already seen in Chapter 3 that this happens in the thoughts, emotions and the will or actions and can be marked by strong feelings. In a certain sense the adolescent experiences a last detachment from the 'childhood-symbiotic relationship' with his parents, which leads to anger, sadness and fear, but also has positive aspects like curiosity, longing, creativity and joy. Awakening sexuality leads these feelings to be expressed in the search for others, often for another form of symbiosis, always paired with the longing for themselves. The questions: Who am I? Where am I going? What is my task in life? Who do I belong to? show us the development of the Adult Ego State. In order to take on the responsibility for themselves, their wishes and actions adolescents need to be nurtured both by the caring and the critical Parent. They also need to develop their own point of view out of their personal values and learn to set themselves their own limits.

Often they go over the top during this process and start acting rebelliously and obstinately in a similar way to a small child. This rebellion of the Child Ego State is often essential to finding oneself. It helps parents to be aware of this fact so that they do not 'fall apart' themselves.

As parents you still need to provide a protective space within which the adolescents can learn to become independent and autonomous. Parents, with their Adult Ego State, can decide when they want to support and relieve their children, and when it is better to let them take on more responsibility. Excessive financial input or washing, ironing and cooking for your children even once they have left home ties the adolescent down. This often leads to expressions like: 'It would be terrible for my mother if she was not allowed to do my washing.'

Parents have to learn to accept that they are not necessarily the most important person in the life of their children anymore, and that their child can have other productive relationships.

During this developmental phase parents increasingly need to treat adolescents as equals. This new relationship quality needs a new form of relationship cultivation, where talking is the basis. It can become a habit in the family to have a kind of family meeting, which not only deals with family conflict but also helps towards consciously observing each other. The free Child Ego State of the parents can emerge in these meetings, when they enjoy the conversations and are curious about meeting their children. As the teenager's ability to observe increases he can also take part in the inner life of his parents, listening to what weighs on their mind or which questions occupy them.

Example: *Mrs B is sitting in the garden by herself when her eighteen-year-old daughter, Carla, comes home. Carla notices by her mother's behaviour that something is not right. In the past this would have irritated her, perhaps she would even have provoked her mother, now she goes up to her: 'Hey, mum, what's wrong?' After her mother does not say much she continues: 'Come on, mum, I have to go back into town anyway, I'll take you with me and we can go and have a cup of coffee.' So it turns out that the afternoon with her daughter was a real help for the mother.*

The child has developed different ego states during the course of his personality development, which enable him to meet other people adequately and appropriately depending on the situation. Naturally the child's development is not restricted to upbringing and socializing alone. Every child also brings an intrinsic nature with him, which reveals itself in his constitution and temperament. But despite this the experiences of early childhood and adolescence, in particular, play a large part in the later life-concept of the child. Upbringing does not only touch the emotional level, but also shapes the brain. Current brain research shows clear correlations in this area. The neurobiologist, Gerald Hüther, and his colleague, Helmut Bonney, a family therapist, stress how strongly educational measures affect the structure of the brain:

> 'All the highly complex networks, which do not happen automatically but are only formed and stabilised when activated and used, could not have developed without many suggestions and encouragement, disciplining and admonishing; that is without the active influence of other people on our brain development. Our brain is structured by these other people and what we have acquired from them to a much greater extent than previously believed.'[34]

Because of this fact different attitudes to life are formed which then influence behaviour during further life. The same is true for social experiences and processes, which can unfortunately also lead children into dead ends where they need our help to find their way out. In this case it is necessary that the adult takes on the responsibility for finding a new way, which can then be followed together with the children. The following description of the four life attitudes according to Thomas A. Harris helps you to assess yourself and possibly realize which 'unfiltered' attitudes children receive.

But first I would like to describe a few exercises that can help parents to observe more closely the development of the different personality parts in their children.

Empathy exercises to help understand the child's personality parts.

Up until six months

You need some time and peace for this exercise!

Lie down comfortably; let yourself sink into whatever you are lying on. Wait until you have become completely calm. Now imagine you have very loving parents; you have just been born and both of them are there for you.

You are lovingly looked after and stroked, you can feel how your back is softly touched and rubbed, careful fingers move over your face, your forehead. Your father says something to you, your mother whispers something into your ear. You cannot understand anything, but you feel content and safe. You are lying completely secure and are protected, everything is done for you, and others think for, and look after, you. The light is dimmed and you are wrapped warmly. All this is done for you just because you are there, how you are.

(After this 'trip' it is advisable to stretch yourself and consciously look around at your familiar surroundings).

This exercise can give you energy and inspiration for how to treat your child and other people important to you.

From six to eighteen months

This exercise is suitable for couples and groups of parents: Sit on the ground and let yourself be blindfolded. Someone else from the group makes sure you do not hurt yourself.

On the ground you are many different objects which you can put into your mouth. Concentrate solely on feeling. How does a stone feel in your hand? Feel its weight, temperature and surface.

What do you experience when you concentrate solely on feeling with your hands and mouth? How do you feel if others think for you, if you do not have to worry about safety und you can just experience?

Exercise for self-observation
For two days, using pen and paper, count how often you say 'No!' to your child.

From eighteen to thirty-six months
This exercise requires peace and some time!

Look for a peaceful place and relax: imagine you are having an argument with your sister or your younger brother, he has broken one of your possessions. You are beside yourself with anger. At home several relatives are visiting, like grandparents, aunts and uncles. Every one of them says something about your anger: what does your father, uncle, grandfather say? What about your mother, aunt, grandmother?
— How do you feel after hearing these things?
— What are your conclusions regarding the feelings of anger and annoyance?
— What do you decide to do in future when you are annoyed?

Exercise for self-observation
During the next days, notice how you react to the annoyance of your small child.
— What does his annoyance release in you?
— What conclusions do you reach because of it?

From three to six years
This exercise is suitable for couples and groups of parents. Sit down together and imagine you are children between the ages of three and six. Use the language of your children, talk about what you like in your family, what you do not like and what you would like.

Then talk about what everyone experienced and how you felt afterwards.

Now imagine that your child is playing 'doctors' with neighbouring children. You can see it from some distance.
— What does your C say?
— What does your P say?
— What does your A say?
— What do the parents of the other children say? And the neighbours?
— What would your parents have said?
— How do you want to react?

From six to twelve years
Take the time to sit down and relax. Think of an argument with your daughter/son who is in this age group: You want to implement something that they don't want. Remember the situation exactly and listen to what you would say internally. Which words do you use (for example, 'you should' or 'you shouldn't')? If you wanted to make a rule, what would it sound like?

In our family I would like ...
In our family I do not want ...
— What does your C say to that?
— What does your P say?
— What does your A say?
— Do you know the traditional rules?

Exercise for self-observation:
Pay attention to what the child does well and how you show you are happy with him. Do not make any other comments about his actions for two days. See whether you are happy with what your child does within the next week.

From thirteen to nineteen years
This exercise requires some time and peace!

Think back to your adolescence and imagine your parting from your parents as if it was happening now.

— How is it for you, and are you well prepared for this step?

— What are the circumstances of your leaving and do your parents support you?

— Do you hold yourself back or let go?

— How do you feel: remember what you did not like and think of what was nice with your parents.

And now imagine your daughter/son wants to leave home. S/he is well prepared for this day. You have given him/her the chance to grow up sheltered in the parental home and act responsibly, develop self-confidence and treat others and themselves well.

— How does this picture make you feel?

You can do this exercise at different times, when the children grow older or when you are having problems with them. Perhaps you will come into contact with important feelings.

The four fundamental life attitudes

Eric Berne has reduced the fundamental maxims of human communication to a short formula: 'I am okay, you are okay,' which means: if I am happy with myself and can accept the other person, then there should not be any problems with communication. But this is an ideal state!

We have seen by the development of the personality parts how strongly the psychological development is dependant on the parent's upbringing. The child does not always feel: 'I am okay — you are okay.' Much more frequently children have the experience that 'I am not okay — you are okay,' due to the use of 'you' messages like 'You always knock everything down,' 'you've dirtied yourself again' and 'Can't you stop doing that?' Or they feel: 'you can be okay if …' Such a little person will try terribly hard to receive tender loving care, and to feel accepted.

Eric Berne differentiates between four basic attitudes as the foundation for the individual position in life:[35]

1. I am okay, you are okay

With this constructive attitude I feel neither superior nor inferior, and due to this do not need to manipulate others nor myself. 'Okay' certainly does not mean that I think that everything that the other person says is good or right. Rather I can admit my own and other's mistakes without devaluing the other or myself as a person. This attitude furthers good communication and effective work. But it is hardly possible — particularly in conflict situations — to preserve it consistently. And there is probably not one person who is solely in this life position.

2. I am okay, you are not okay

This position, which Berne calls paranoid, arrogant or projective, results from an unrealistic feeling of power and superiority. Usually a basically unstable self-esteem hides behind this stance. People with this basic attitude like to take on tasks ('I can do it better anyway!'). They usually give others or 'circumstances' the blame for failure. A fundamental aspect of this behaviour is that any possibly existing shortcomings in the abilities of other people are always linked to a degradation of the person. The fact that many people have great difficulties in accepting criticism may show how widespread this position is.

3. I am not okay, you are okay

People with this attitude feel subjectively overwhelmed and often take on all the blame. They often start statements with self-devaluation, in connection to super-elevating the abilities of others. 'Can I ask a really stupid question?' or: 'But I definitely can't express that as well as you!' Here too individual abilities and competences are inappropriately related to the person as a whole. In this case Berne talks about the depressive stance.

4. I am not okay, you are not okay

This inner attitude is related to the feeling of a deep lack of goal and purpose in life. These people cannot see anything positive about themselves or others. They often appear cynical and tend towards treating constructive and positive solutions with irony or degradation. This attitude is sometimes used as a 'relief' from the preceding position. ('I am useless, but I will prove that others are also not normal'). If a person remains in this stance for a longer period then it can become a danger for body and psyche.

These life stances, frequently in alternation, can contribute towards a disturbed behavioural pattern. It is helpful to remember that during childhood such patterns of behaviour can sometimes be sensible, creative and often quite literally essential for survival. But as adults, parents and educators it is advantageous to take a new look at these positions, as often old suppositions are no longer correct and the resulting conflicts perhaps not appropriate for us anymore. As educators and examples for children we carry the responsibility for what we confront them with, both consciously and unconsciously, as this in turn influences their own life concept. There is no doubt that this task is difficult and cannot succeed all the time, but our children are thankful for each new attempt.

Basic transaction patterns

Eric Berne chose the term 'transaction analysis' to highlight the fact that exchange between people is the main emphasis of this communication theory. We have seen that transaction analysis is based on the Ego State model. It offers a clear way of describing and making conscious communication between people. The word 'transaction' describes the smallest complete communication unity comprising a stimulus (a comment, a question, a facial expression etc.) and its reaction; it encompasses all verbal and non-verbal aspects of communication. Thus one conversation is composed of many different transactions between the single Ego States of the participants.

Berne differentiates three basic patterns of transactions:

- Complementary (parallel) transactions;
- Crossed transactions;
- Covert transactions.

The following examples can help you understand the different transactions and make your own communication more conscious.

Complementary transactions

Most of our daily communication consists of this kind of transaction. One of the mother's ego states appeals to a specific ego state of the child. If the child accepts this 'invitation' and reacts with the ego state spoken to, then a complementary transaction results. This allows the conversation to flow, as expectations and reactions of the conversation partners correspond to each other.

Mother: 'Eliza, can you tidy up your room, please?'
Eliza: 'Yes, I'll do it in a minute:'

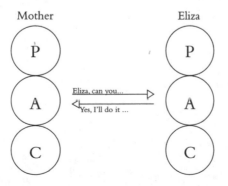

Father: 'Jon, your tools are lying around on the workbench again.'

Jonas: 'Oh, sorry, I didn't mean to leave them there.'

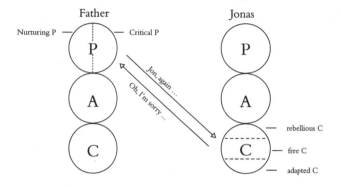

Granny: 'I would really like to play cards with you.'

Grandchildren: 'Great, we also want to play:'

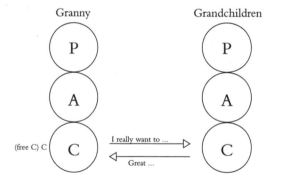

Mother: 'Are you going to be quiet soon?!'

Children: 'Huh, silly old goat, we always have to be quiet!'

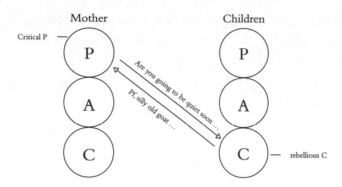

Crossed transactions

If a discussion takes an unexpected turn, so that irritations result, we have a crossed transaction, that is, the child does not react with the ego state the mother has appealed to. Usually a short period of confusion or a break follows, which sometimes also leads to termination of the conversation. The course of such a conversation can often end completely different than planned.

Mother: 'Mona, have done your homework?'
Mona. 'What does my homework actually have to do with you!'

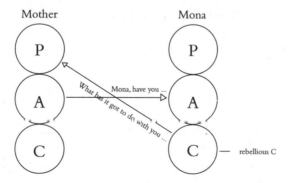

Father: 'Olga, shall I help you with your homework?'
Olga: 'Oh, don't say you've suddenly got time for me!'

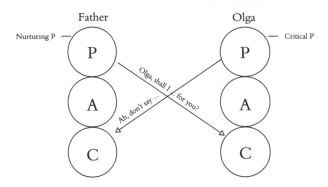

These kinds of transactions and conversations are well known to many people, as they lead to annoyance, confusion, disappointment and other bad feelings. But there is also a way out, by productively crossing the crossed transactions. By consciously using the crossed transaction I can invite the other person to leave their unproductive path, change their ego state and to continue with something constructive.

In this case the dialogue between the fourteen-year-old Mona and her mother could end like this:

Mother: 'Mona, have you done your homework?'

Mona: 'What does my homework actually have to do with you?!'

Mother: 'What do you mean by that?'

Mona: 'I mean that I can think of my homework myself, and your question annoys me because I get the impression that you don't trust me to do it.'

Mother: 'I would like to talk to you about that in more detail again.'

Mona: 'Yes, okay, that is probably a good idea.'

The mother's consciously employed question, what Mona actually means, causes both of them transfer to the adult Ego State, with gives the conversation an informative turn.

Covert transactions

These transactions happen when a further, covert level is added to the apparently obvious conversation level. The former is also called the psychological level, the latter the social level. The actual message is not expressed directly or at all, but has to be inferred indirectly by the sound of the voice, the intonation, the facial expression or a memory of previous situations. The statement itself is on a psychological level, which means that the emotional outcome of the conversation will also be on this level. Children are often forced to learn to read between the lines from an early age, as they soon realize this is where the real message lies. Two level transactions often lead to confusion and entanglement in the conversation. An attentive ear helps to notice these transactions early on and put a stop to them.

Father: 'Matthias, have you set the table?'
Mathias: 'Yes, why?'
Father: 'Oh, nothing, I was just asking.' (meanwhile he is rearranging the cutlery as he appears to be unsatisfied with how it has been set, but he doesn't say anything.)

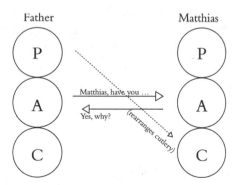

Exercises

• Get to know yourself in your different ego states, also your non-verbal expressions like gestures, facial expression and pitch:

— Child Ego State: particularly its vulnerable parts, fears and the most common way it expresses its feelings,
— Parent Ego State: its commands and prohibitions, its unshake-able principles,
— Adult Ego State: its protective measures like maintaining eye contact, anticipating and assessing a situation, being able to put oneself in the other's shoes, making agreements and sticking to them.

• Which of your ego states do you use to communicate with your family more often, or not so often?
• Imagine a person with whom you often have problems and one with whom you get on well. Try to observe which ego states the person concerned uses with you. With which ego states do you react? How much are your productive ego states (nurturing Parent, Adult and free Child) involved?
• To find out even more about your inner and outer transactions I would like to recommend writing a 'logbook': Think of a current problem and sketch, write down and organize   everything you can think of concerning the different ego states. For the next step your Adult can evaluate the different aspects. Perhaps you will notice that some of the ego states never get a look in. How can you give them a part in retrospect? What have you found out about yourself during this process?

Transactions in day-to-day family life

Last summer I spent a week's holiday at the North Sea with my children. On the beach we sat in a large beach chair like all the other summer guests. This 'retreat in the midst of many people gave everyone a private sphere, in which they could be at home. During this week three different families were based around me, who naturally gave me insight into their family lives.

Family A

This family was comprised of a father and his two children; the daughter was about six years old, the younger brother about four. Typical of this family was a loud, cutting tone of voice, with which commands and threats were expressed at every possible moment. The father wanted his peace, the children on the other hand wanted his help with building a sandcastle.

Daughter: 'Daddy, can you help us with the digging? I want to make a big sandcastle'

Father: 'Oh no, surely you can do it by yourself.'

Brother: 'I can help you:'

Sister: 'No, you always break everything!'

Father: 'Just let him help you, you're always so troublesome!'

Daughter: 'No I'm not, you're troublesome!'

Father: 'If you don't that stop that right now I'll get angry and then I'll make you play with him!'

His mobile phone rings, and he telephones with commitment. During this time the children fight about the spade, the father barks out commands while continuing to phone: 'Now stop it, can't you behave for once?' He continues phoning for nearly half an hour. Meanwhile children from the neighbouring beach chairs have joined them to help. The same scene repeated itself with slight variations every day.

Family B

This family was comprised of a mother with three children aged four, six and seven. When they moved into their beach chair each child had a backpack and together they carried a rubber dinghy. The children unpacked their treasures and started playing. The mother gave them a helpful hint by drawing a line in the sand to show them how far away they could go from the beach basket, and then lay down in the rubber dinghy — where she had a little nap! The tone of voice in this family was warm and benevolently supportive. Here too conflicts arose during play. The children built themselves a house with a kitchen in their sandy hollow, where they cooked with shells, sticks and seaweed. But now they couldn't agree on what to cook, the youngest one argued with his brother.

Four-year old: 'I don't want to have spinach, I don't like it!'

Seven-year old: 'Come on, I'll cook you some carrots, you're sure to like them.'

Six-year old: 'I'll make pudding.'

The three of them were intensely occupied with making the menu, and were talking together very loudly. The mother seemed to think it was a bit too loud for the other guests (or perhaps for herself). She went up to the children and asked them quietly and nicely if they could turn down their kitchen radio. Without opposition, one of the children said: 'yes, okay!' and they continued cooking until their mother was called for lunch. They were just going to start when the four-year old said quietly to his mother. 'But mummy, we haven't said grace yet.' Quietly they said grace together. The next day I was nearly lucky enough to be invited for lunch.

Family C

A mother, a father, an eight-year-old daughter, and ten and twelve-year-old sons. This family did not have a beach chair, they had brought blankets and a wind break. Everything was built up respectfully and they arranged themselves cosily. As I always turned our beach chair to face the sun I had family C in my field of vision in the afternoon. They were noticeably quiet. The mother lay in the sun, the father drank his beer and looked towards the mudflats. The eight year old listened to a tape, while the ten and twelve year olds played with a game boy. They did not speak much together and when they did it was only single words or mumbled sentences like: 'Just leave me in peace'.

Now you might ask: well, dear Mrs Kiel-Hinrichsen, what did your family transaction look like? Here you are!

Family D

A mother with two children, a ten-year-old daughter and a twelve-year-old son, move into their beach chair for a week. They are also weighed down with spades, ball games and kites.

First all of they sit quietly quite overtaxed by all the people and impressions and look at each other. Together they then discuss who gets a seat in the beach chair at what time; for an emergency they have brought their own small beach chair. Everyone agrees on a walk through the mud flats. Things become a bit difficult with the twelve-year-old in regard to applying sun lotion, but reason prevails!

After the walk the mother needs a break, which both children accept, they had already decided during the walk that they wanted to dig themselves into the mud.

Suddenly the two children are standing in front of their mother as she awakens from her short nap, covered from head to foot in mud. Still slightly dazed she rants: 'My goodness, did you have to make yourself so dirty, the tide isn't coming back for another two hours.'

Thank goodness neither of them took it too seriously, but as competent children countered: 'But we can go and have a shower.'

A few moments later the mother was able to be happy about the naturalness and freedom of them both.

Exercise

If it joyfully and creatively appeals to your inner free child then draw graphically the transactions of the different families and, as a second step, think of more creative solutions. A third step could be that you write and draw your own family transactions.

If others do not answer your love with love,
Examine your own kindness.
If others do not respond to your attempt to lead them
  with order,
Examine your own wisdom.
If others do not reply to your politeness,
Examine your own consideration.
In other words,
Examine yourself whenever you do not reach your target.

Meng-tzu (Mencius)

8. Education Towards a 'Whole Human Being'

Education of the senses and social abilities

You may well ask yourself what education of the senses has to do with social abilities, but a healthy physical and emotional development is the foundation for good social abilities and conflict management. Caring for the senses is one of the pillars of our human existence, which is comparable to the growing roots of a plant and its later flower. The better the ground and the care, the more magnificent the flower. The same is true for sense impressions; they are the finest 'nourishment' for the child. Just as we can live off tinned food, which does not build a strong body, we can also 'fill' ourselves and our children with low quality, or even damaging sense impressions. This can lead to impairment in perceptive abilities, for example, not being able to listen well. Because of this I would like to look at the sense theory in greater detail later in this chapter.

In general there are five human senses that are recognized, although for quite some time modern research has found that we use more senses for perception.

Rudolf Steiner speaks of twelve senses. In his teachings of the senses he describes how the spiritual world works in the human being through the sense organism. We can think of the human being as an image of the macrocosm. If one wants to visualize how the spiritual and the sense organism affect each other it is helpful to consider the following picture: imagine that the human consciousness moves through the twelve senses like the sun in the sky moves through the zodiac signs by day and night. We have senses which we can call night senses, they are not part of our consciousness but work subconsciously within us; they register an objective occurrence within their own organism.

They are called the *lower senses*, the *bodily, will* or *basal senses*.
These are the
- Sense of touch
- Sense of movement
- Sense of life
- Sense of balance

As we emerge from the subconscious and turn towards the outside world, external perceptions develop by encountering the outer world of objects, but at the same time these senses are more 'subjectively' coloured. We have moved from the night senses to the dawn senses.
- Sense of smell
- Senses of taste
- Sense of sight
- Sense of temperature

These senses are mediators between the self and the outside world, therefore they are called *medial, environment* or *feeling senses*.

They lead us to the day senses in which we are completely awake, completely conscious.
- Sense of hearing or sound
- Sense of speech or physiognomy
- Thinking or thought sense
- I-sense

These senses are also called the *upper senses* or the *knowledge senses*.

All the senses convey to us an impression, a perception. No single sense ever works alone, but often three or four work together.

The senses described are gateways for our perceptions:
1. Through the first gateway we receive perceptions of our physical body;
2. Through the second gateway we receive perceptions towards the world;
3. Through the third gateway we receive perceptions towards social understanding, towards the I and You.

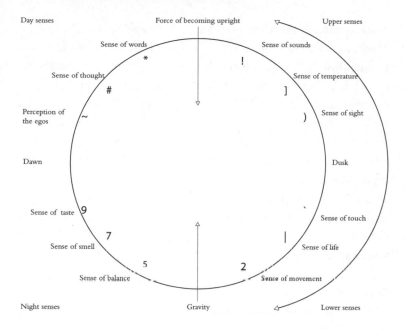

As in many other areas one can think of the human being as an image of the macrocosm: the human consciousness appears in sensory perceptions like the sun in the day and night sky and the different zodiac signs. Our emotions move through the twelve senses just like the sun moves through the twelve zodiac signs.

Introduction to the teaching of the senses

As I cannot, and do not want to, assume that all readers know about the meaning and range of the twelve senses, I will describe their essence in the following sections.

The four lower senses, basal sense, will sense

Sense of touch

The sense of touch is found in a tension between inner and outer perceptive organs: although we touch the outer world with it, it transmits an 'inner' experience. The sense of touch is

spread over the entire body's surface. It experiences the whole
body and its boundaries with everything that does not belong to
it. Each touch the child receives transmits a feeling of the self to
the child, whether it is through physical contact and daily care
or through contact with clothes and shoes, with which in turn
the child connects to the ground, or in relation to the elements
water and air. This leads her to elementary experiences of herself
and the world, of the 'own' and the 'foreign.' This can be seen
beautifully when small children go for a walk with their parents
and after a short time whine: 'Mummy, daddy — arm!' Here we
often find nothing else expressed other than the longing for a
sense of themselves in the big world (as opposed to the smaller
world at home).

Sense of life

With our sense of life we experience ourselves as a living being,
which fills the space of our body. The feeling of the sense of life
remains unconscious, its perceptive organ is the autonomic nervous system. It has the task to perceive the current state of our
organs and metabolism. Karl König compared the sense of life to
a thin curtain that shows the inner climate, like a barometer of the
life processes.[36] During well-being this remains still, while it starts
moving when the body feels hunger, thirst, tiredness, pain etc.
The small child's sense of life is not yet linked solely to her own
physicality, but rather is still extended to include the outer world.
If she has hurt herself she does not necessarily feel the pain in
her own body, but more in the cause as, for example, the branch,
which has made the 'sore' bit.

The sense of life is also called well-being, vital or health
sense. Without the feeling of an inner well-being the small child
becomes whiny, difficult to motivate and also often does not
progress cognitively. We will see later in which way this sense is
related to the development of thinking.

All pleasant skin sensations work on the sense of life. Bathing,
showering, massages and particularly also handling natural materials that still carry life quality (for example, acorns, chestnuts etc.)

or playing with sand and baking bread stimulate this sense. It then conveys contentment and a feeling of harmony.[37]

Sense of movement

The sense of movement is a different case entirely: imagine a growing plant or a lower, immobile animal and compare it to an animal that can move around freely. This gives us an idea of the sense of movement, which increasingly awakens during the child's development. The organ of the sense of movement is the motor nervous system of the spinal cord and central nervous system. Twenty nerve pairs come out of the spinal cord, which let us feel movement. We are not conscious of the movement itself, only of the sensation which occurs in us by the movement. The sense of movement can be imagined as a large string instrument, where the movements play their melodies, harmonies and rhythms.

We can differentiate between four areas of movement:

- Gross motor activity from which we receive a feeling for large movements;
- Fine motor activity which transfers the feeling for small movements;
- Rotational motor activity from which we experience the feeling of the rotation of hand, foot and head; and
- Delicate motor activity, which we experience when our eyes move while looking and when our jaw, tongue and lips move while speaking.

Particularly nowadays, with our extreme lack of movement, children are dependant on differentiated suggestions from parents, kindergarten and school to develop their sense of movement. This is one of the elementary senses and later gives us the basis for our feeling of freedom.

Sense of balance

The sense of balance is last of the basal senses. It a specific human quality, as no animal has it in the same way. The sense of balance transmits the feeling of inner peace. It is located in the inner ear and makes us conscious of our current position and movement in space, gives us the feeling of being in equilibrium and experiencing our own gravity as a resting place.

The child attains the sense of balance in its first year of life. 'Through its upright position it trains the sense of balance, with enables it to think and mature into human uprightness.'[38] During the following years it is necessary to give the sense of balance differentiated stimulation to help the human being attain physical and emotional stability. Through Rudolf Steiner's teaching of the senses we know about the strong relationship of the sense of balance to the sense of hearing; both organs lie close together in the head. Many difficulties in upbringing are caused by children who are not sufficiently calm internally and consequently do not listen properly. This will continue to occupy us in the following chapters.

To sum up I would like to emphasize that these four basal senses are the foundation for a healthy existential sensation of the body and lead to the feelings of *trust, well-being, freedom* and *peace* — an essential basis for later social abilities.

The four central senses — environmental senses — sensation senses

While the lower senses give us a feeling for our own body, the central senses transmit perceptual sensations offered by the outer world. Caring for the *senses of smell, taste, sight* and *temperature* establishes an existential feeling in the psyche. We sense the warm sun, cool wind or cold sea water with our sense of temperature. We smell sweet smelling hay, manure on the field, perfume or baked bread with our sense of smell. Through our tongue, the organ of the sense of taste, we receive sweet, sour, bitter and salty sensations. These senses awaken strong feelings of sympathy and antipathy. Food that elicits aversion, or wholesome smells, can trigger the strongest feelings of disgust and well-being. The relationship between these senses and feelings can be seen linguistically in expressions like: 'That is a matter of taste,' 'she is a sour old woman,' 'the bitter truth,' 'a tasteless person,' 'spice up my life.'

The *sense of sight* is different from the other senses in several ways. The eye can be seen as the most sensitive and mobile organ. It is in continuous movement and is a perceptive organ of the I in action. What happens in the eye during the act of seeing makes it possible for us to be present with our I, our consciousness.

Here too we often express our emotions through words referring to the sense of sight, for example: 'I feel blue,' or 'I can see red.'

Emotions are revealed by the look in the eye. The eye can speak, smile, wound, express feelings like love, hatred and compassion. Human resolve becomes visible in the eye.

The *sense of temperature* is the gateway from the central senses to the higher senses. The experience of warmth or cold at specific points on the skin happens because the thermo-receptors in the skin are stimulated. But no specific organ is responsible for the sense of temperature in general — the person as a whole feels the sensation. Warmth perception can only happen when the warmth coming from outside is met by an emotional sensation, which leads to feelings of opening up and relaxation. But the opposite can also be true: if the outer environment is emotionally cold, this can have physical effects. The surroundings, so to speak, draws off the warmth of the person, who starts to 'freeze emotionally,' and, particularly with small children, physically. The sense of emotional warmth and cold, as well as feelings towards other people, are also expressed linguistically: we describe some people as 'emotionally cold' or 'warm hearted,' speak of 'glowing admirer,' of 'cold calculation,' a 'cool undertone' or say 'I feel warm in my heart' etc.

The basic characteristic of this group of senses can be summed up again: the central senses give the human being an emotional existential feeling!

The four higher senses; knowledge senses, social senses

Sense of hearing

The ear is the primary sense organ of the human being. In the embryo the ear is developed as the first sense a few days after conception. The sense of hearing is the earliest sense, and is also the last one to leave the person, as the ear continues to hear as long as the soul is still connected to the body.

Hearing leads us from the outside to inside, it gives us a feeling which can be described as 'I am here.' Noises in general give us a feeling of existence, they can be organized into sounds, voices and tones.

A range of different processes happen when we hear speech. The information transferred from the auditory nerve to the brain section above, the temporal lobe, breaks down into different perceptive fields. There are areas of the brain that only transfer volume and pitch etc., but also others that enable us to register the voice tone and musicality of speech. Other areas again help us to understand the meaning of speech. There are at least three sense organs which participate when we hear speech:

- The sense of hearing alone, with which we perceive all kinds of sound and noises;
- The sense of words, with which we recognize the sounds of speech and the words as such;
- The sense of thoughts, with which we recognize what the speaker means in relation to the circumstances.

The sense of hearing, also called *tone sense,* is the sense with the greatest reception.

The highest possible alertness of the child is achieved when he hears tones. The sounds he hears penetrates his entire organism. *The ear always hears, even if attention is directed towards other perceptions and actions.* This is a good place to listen to one's surroundings and consciously perceive which sounds educate towards not listening, and which towards hearing.

Sense of speech

The sense of words or speech is already present in a newborn, but is not yet functional. The sense of speech is only sensitized by the interaction between the speech centre in the brain and the developing motor organism, as well as by the imitation of people's facial expressions and articulation and listening to sounds. *The spoken word requires a calm, listening ear and a relaxed body!*

The ability to speak is stimulated precisely by this calm listening reflecting on the inside (ether body) of the child. We can understand this better if we remember that the sense of speech and the sense of movement are closely related: our entire motor organism is at the same time a sense organism for perceiving words. It is only because we keep our body still while listening that we can understand the spoken words.[39] If we do not speak the words internally while reading then the text cannot be understood. But by keeping still and not letting the 'inner motion' be acted 'outside,' sense and visualization of the word arises.

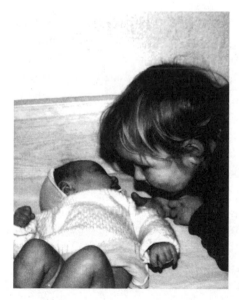

By listening to the sounds of its surroundings or being spoken to as directly as possible the small child gradually develops a sense of understanding words.

Sense of thought

This sense develops in parallel with speech development. It gives the child an awareness of the structure and content of other people's thoughts.

A small child is still very sensitive to the thoughts of the people around him. Long before he can understand them he takes in the emotional content even if it is not spoken aloud. Perceptions of the sense of thought penetrate into the inner organs, which can then be expressed through screaming, stomach-ache etc. Parents having a partnership crisis sometimes wonder why their child also becomes disagreeable, making the situation more difficult.

The relationship of the sense of thought to one of the lower senses can clarify its particular quality: the sense of thought develops as a consequence of the sense of life's activity in childhood. The child perceives the coherence of his organ functions and also the coherence of the sequence of actions in his surroundings, and these impressions shape the central neural networks throughout the years. They then become the sense organ for understanding the thoughts of other people.[40]

Sense of I

Rudolf Steiner called the perceptive organ for the other person's I the 'sense of I.' As it always concerns the other person, one should really talk about the 'sense of you.' When we hear another person talking, we perceive more than just the sound of their voice, the melody of the sentences and the thought content of the spoken words. We perceive the other person as a distinctive person with our sense of I.

The first stirring of the sense of I can be compared to the perception of a fleeting shadow. One can also say: just as a colour has an effect on us through the medium of our eye, so the I of the other affects us through our sense of I. This is the transformation of a basal sense, the sense of touch. The sense of touch is a mediating sense for the sense of I in childhood. During this stage every physical encounter is simultaneously an emotional meeting, an I-you-encounter.

> During the course of childhood the sense of I
> gradually detaches itself from the sense of touch.
> The sense of touch becomes de-souled, as it were
> [...] The sense of I is continuously liberated from
> the need to touch. From this point we can expe-
> rience the other person in its uniqueness, without
> having to hug it first. This gives us the chance to
> use our I sense increasingly as a liberated 'culture
> sense' [...] The independence of the sense of I
> awakens, which is necessary for social abilities in
> later life:[41]

The sense of touch in the small child unconsciously also
encompasses the experience of the essence of the human. This
naturally leads to connections in the nervous system, which in
turn develops the sense of I. The single developmental phases
are described below:

- Pre-stage   first smile
- 6 months   rejecting strangers
- 3 years   I
- 7 years   I strengthening
- 9 years   beginning of sense of I
- 12 years   sense of I strengthening
- 21 years   full inner maturity

To summarize, one can say that the four higher senses lead to emotions which enable a healthy existence in spiritual actions. Listening
allows emotions to transfer from external visible space to an inner
space, from where they can connect to thinking inspiration.

At the beginning of this section we likened the development
of the twelve senses to the growth of a plant. The lower senses
constitute the roots, the central senses the stalk with the leaves
and the higher senses the upwardly-striving blossom — we can
experience the plant in its entirety. And just as plants are capable
of metamorphosis, we can look at the metamorphosis within
the human senses:

- The sense of hearing is the transformed sense of balance;
- The sense of word or speech is a transformed sense of movement;
- The sense of thoughts is the transformed sense of life;
- The sense of I is a transformation of the sense of touch.

The better the ground has been prepared for the roots, the will senses, the healthier and more colourful the blossom will be, the senses of knowledge. I would like to call them *social senses*.

> 'Let us not forget that every social living together, that a future culture needs to be directly founded on the cultivation of the senses of knowledge, but that these sense organs in turn can only develop properly when all the other senses, when the entire sense organism of the human being has been properly cared for through education and self-education.'[42]

Lack of sense experiences and their compensation

> *Out of himself the human being cannot experience*
> *Any higher sense than the central senses.*
> Rudolf Steiner[43]

Perceptive difficulties or impairments occur when a child does not receive enough sense impressions, whether out of himself or because of his environment, or because he does not have any social examples by which to develop positive sense impressions. This becomes obvious particularly with regard to social abilities.

Michaela Glöckler has found succinct connections in this area:

> Perception impairments and a lack of empathy are always also signs that particular experiences and abilities have not been acquired. Where there is a

lack of empathy for the world, there is as a rule
a corresponding impairment in the creation of a
healthy self-awareness.[44]

Impairments	Consequences
In the sense of touch	Lack of trust in the self and world
In the sense of life	Lack of a sense of harmony and sense of experience, cannot be bothered doing things
In the sense of movement	Lack of a sense of freedom
In the sense of balance	Lack of the chance to find inner peace
In the sense of smell	Lack of a differentiated dealing with emotions of sympathy and antipathy
In the sense of taste	Tendency to judge only according to personal taste. One is used to ones favourite food and has not learnt to taste extensively enough
In the sense of sight	Lack of inner far-sightedness (soul blindness)
In the sense of temperature	Lack of inner warmth and attentiveness
In the sense of hearing	Lack of inwardness
In the sense of words	Lack of individual understanding of expression for forms, gestures and words. Also lack of word conscientiousness
In the sense of thought	Lack of understanding of connections, tendency to misunderstandings
In the sense of I	Lack of experiences of beings, of sense of reality[45]

Even if you notice impairment tendencies in yourself or your child, all is not lost. The metamorphosis of the senses can show what can help. Take a look at the twelve senses in a linear development from the inner senses to the outer sense (see diagram opposite)

> When a sense organ directed towards the inside develops, then a sense organ is simultaneously developed directed towards the outside — comparable to the laws of weighing scales. So you can see that not only do the basal senses transform into the higher social and knowledge senses, but such transformations also happen in the centre senses: from the sense of smell to the sense of temperature, from the sense of taste to the sense of sight. Between the latter two there is a resting point, called 'Hypomochlion' by Rudolf Steiner. This knowledge is of great consequence for therapeutic treatment in curative education [but also in pedagogy and parental upbringing, M.K-H.].'[46]

The diagram opposite clarifies the relations of the different senses to each other. It shows, for example, that paying attention to the sense of touch in a child with a disturbed sense of I can work in a healing way. This is not only true for children — it also applies to exhausted mothers with a dimmed perception of their children, who can particularly benefit from attentiveness in this area, for example, through massages.

This makes it clear why one cannot think so well during illness, tiredness or hunger and why one then often has difficulties understanding. Once the need is eased or the illness improved, then the ability to perceive immediately changes again.

By looking at relationships between the senses we can discover how to indirectly stimulate a deficient perception. If, for example, your children do not like eating, then you can remember that the eye eats too, and become more creative in

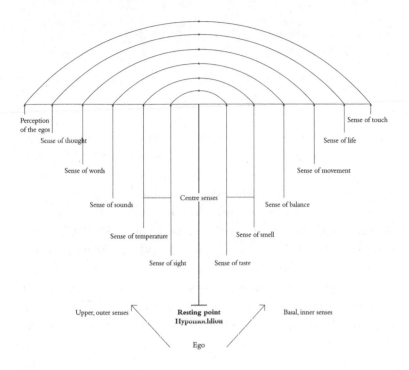

There are close relationships between the individual senses: each inner sense corresponds to an outer sense. If one wants to have a positive effect on one of the outer senses, then it can be helpful to look after the respective inner sense.

presenting the meals. This might mean fewer verbal negotiations. Or pay attention to times when you or your child is particularly sensitive to smells, and think about whether that could have anything to do with physical coldness, as then warmth helps!

And what if you have a child who cannot or will not listen properly ,,.? This phenomenon will be looked at in more detail in the following chapter.

What does the development of the senses have to do with the ability to listen?

During children's upbringing the foundations are laid
For listening or not listening.

In his teachings of the senses Rudolf Steiner describes the close relationship of the sense of balance and the sense of hearing. Both organs lie close together in the temporal bone of the skull. Everyone knows how difficult it is to listen when one is not calm inside. The example of Josefa and Antonella, at the start of this book, showed this quite clearly (page 15). Josefa could neither concentrate on the phone call with her friend, nor get involved with Antonella's needs as she felt torn within herself.

There are at least three senses which are involved when we hear and understand speech: the sense of hearing, the sense of words, with which we recognize the sounds of speech and words, and the sense of thought, with which we understand the content of words. The sense of I is of great importance for children, as they can and want to perceive the other person as an individual being. In my view this can be seen in a double sense, as what does the child want to meet? They want to meet an adult who is in command of all their senses if they are interested in the child. All too often this is not the case for parents and educators when we are dealing with children. Particularly with regard to children many of us have the habit of saying important things 'by the by,' often without even looking at the person we are speaking to. If we remember that the small child needs the sense of touch for her development and to sense herself, then we are nearing the truth of the key words of communication: 'it is only with the heart that one can see rightly.'

Because:
Children can hear when:
• We devote ourselves directly to them;
• We help them to remain balanced;
• If necessary we touch them physically;

- We touch them emotionally;
- We look at them (this is also touch in a wider sense);
- Our thoughts are concerned with the matter;
- We have used the right tone of voice;
- We criticize the matter, but not the person.

Children can hear when:
- They are not hungry or tired;
- They have a good physical sense foundation; that means if:
  - They experience touch again and again;
  - They can learn varied, different movements;
  - They are stimulated or strengthened in their life energy
  - They can experience sense relationships;
  - They can practise their physical balance;
  - They have learnt to listen;
  - They can imitate the world in play;
  - They feel taken seriously;
  - *They are allowed to be children!*

If they are allowed to be children — this means that we adults have to meet the children where they are in their development and have to treat them in an age-appropriate way.

ADHD children and hearing

In his description of the 'hyperactive child' Gerald Hüther mentions that ADHD children, particularly the younger ones, seemingly 'hear badly.'[47] The spoken words of their parents have so little effect on some of them that a physical hearing disorder is even suspected, which is actually only rarely the case. Parents complain that their child is disobedient. Small children who are able to speak do not appear to want to listen. Their parents are driven to frustration and desperation because their children 'let the information go in one ear and out the other.' They repeat their verbal demands and attempt to reach their child by increasing their volume. This leads to a vicious circle where finally both the parents and the child feel badly treated. Both react with withdrawal from the situation: the child by continuing her actions in a seemingly unrelated manner, the responsible adults by giving up their efforts towards constructive contact. In this case therapeutic counselling can help parents and children to feel addressed and understood and able to act in relation to each other. Once these children can be reached verbally, they start to react appropriately and reliably.

Science has given 'the 'hearing problem' of ADHD children a lot of attention. In fact changes to the central processing of sounds can be shown. According to the results of recent electro-physiological research, small and primary-school children with ADHD problems differ in their auditory receptive functions, which restricts their ability to maintain their attention. This means they do not have a hearing disorder. Children need the so-called entire sensory experience to be able to be able to express themselves in a socially appropriate way. Parents tend to favour a predominantly verbal type of upbringing from an early age, despite its failure, and regardless of the clinically impressive and neurologically verifiable acoustic perceptive variations, thus making it more difficult for the child to perceive the safe rules and limits.[48]

Gerald Hüther, in an interview with the magazine *Der Spiegel*, answers the question of the enormous increase in numbers of ADHD children in relation to the fact that parents are increasingly unsure about the upbringing of their children. In earlier times very strict social circumstances like religion or class gave constraints that also shaped the frontal lobe — and the personality of the child. Nowadays, these constraints have become more or less obsolete and everything seems possible in upbringing. Increasingly parents do not know how to deal with their children.

How should parents, who do not feel sure about their own role, pay loving attention to the needs of particularly sensitive children? Gerald Hüther calls for parental schools, in which parents can learn the most important basic rules — for example 'simple' things like setting limits and giving children new tasks.

> A good mother will make sure that her child always has new problems, and then help it to solve them itself. Only then can the frontal lobe develop optimally [...] Children hold us up a mirror with their behavioural disturbances. In it we can see that we are doing something wrong, if we do not understand that the development of the child's brain does not happen by itself.'[49]

The following suggestions towards training the child's senses should be thought of as a contribution to the requirements set by Gerald Hüther.

Suggestions and exercises for training children's twelve senses

Sense of touch

- Children who do not have a good feeling for themselves benefit from having a large doll, possibly filled with sand. The weight of the doll helps them to obtain a feeling of their own body
- Possibly use heavy blankets for the bed, which 'make a boundary' around the child
- Carry the child in your arms every now and again
- Use clothes made out of different natural materials, this sensitizes the skin
- Provide the child with varied touch experiences by giving her natural substances
- Stimulations of the skin through sponges, a brush which visits the child as a hedgehog etc.
- Touching games, like drawing or doing a maths problem onto their back

- Feeling things placed under a cloth, both with hands and with feet

Providing touch perceptions further away:
- Retrieving balls, marbles, chestnuts from under furniture with a broomstick
- Playing pat the pan
- Walking beside a fence with a stick

Providing perceptions of the self
- Give the child different opportunities to touch himself (finger games, pat-a-cake, crossing the arms over the chest, folding the hands …)

Sense of life
- Any kind of bodily care stimulates the sense of life (cleaning teeth, washing hands, applying creams, cutting nails, combing hair)
- Bathing, showering, splashing, swimming
- Baking
- As well as any kind of emotional attention

Sense of movement
- Support the skilfulness of the child, learn to control movements (for example, by pouring water or tea into jugs and glasses)
- Ball games, also against a wall
- Practise hand and finger dexterity (for example, tying bows; if possible avoid Velcro fastenings)
- Practise hand-eye co-ordination (for example, following alternative hands lying over each other with the eyes)
- Wind balls of wool, plait things, use an embroidery frame, knit a doll, use a weaving loom
- Form and mould modelling substances, from clay to beeswax (sense of temperature)
- Grasp marbles with toes

- Draw with thick crayons using feet
- Finger games, etc, see sense of touch
- Eurythmy, therapeutic riding, work therapy to stimulate the psychomotor
- Stimulate all the mouth movements (give pointed kisses, lick around the mouth and up to the nose ...)

Sense of balance
- The sense of balance is stimulated through pressure and massage
- Stimulation for pregnant people and babies: rocking chair, cradle, hammock
- Swinging, jumping on a trampoline, walking on stilts, pedalos
- Balancing rice and sand sacks on the head
- Climbing trees and on logs
- Juggling balls and cloths
- Playing circus
- Skipping with a rope, hopscotch, skipping on one leg
- Roller skating and ice skating
- Riding a bike (without stabilizers)
- Cutting paper
- Building with small blocks, but also with chairs and larger pieces of wood ...

Sense of smell
- Give children various true-to-life experiences of smell: cow shed, hay harvest, smell of wood in a joinery, potatoes in a fire, soap suds when washing, blooming flowers, mown grass, rotting leaves
- Baking with yeast, the smell out of the oven stimulates the sense of smell
- Washing doll's clothes
- Sanding wood
- Drying fruit
- Making candles (particularly beeswax)
- Sewing small aromatic herb bags

Sense of taste
- A small child still tastes with its entire body and then begins to 'eat with the soul'
- Give children the chance to try out different things, sweet, salty, sour, bitter tastes
- Children are motivated by their eyes, their eye eats too!
- Short stories, in which the children are allowed to taste different things
- Mother and child games, the doll is allowed to try something, the doll's mother too
- Playing shop with different utensils

Sense of sight
- Keep eye contact with the child!
- Do not use a push chair where the child cannot see her mother
- Let the child move in the sunlight in nature
- Light, colourfully painted rooms
- Look at beautiful, child appropriate, picture books
- Draw with water colours and good coloured crayons
- Moveable toys and picture books

Sense of temperature
- Stimulating the sense of temperature in small children also stimulates the brain
- Warm bath water, warm swimming pool
- Kneading warm dough when baking cakes
- Let them touch warm and cold things
- Essential oils to rub in
- Moist-warm stomach wraps for difficulties falling asleep
- Emotional warmth through the higher senses

Sense of hearing
- Avoid background noises!
- Playing hiding games which stimulate listening
- Whisper to the child now and again

- Playing in the play corner while the dolls are sleeping
- Hearing games with closed eyes: paper rustling, ticking clocks, water noises
- Echoes, for example, calling into the milk jug
- Tuning fork, guitar chords
- Playing blind man's bluff as a hearing game

Sense of words
- Set an example through natural, but well articulated speech
- Care of gross and fine motor activity
- Games in a circle, hand and finger games
- Eurythmy for children

Sense of thought
- The child's developing sense of thought is highly sensitive to the thoughts of her surroundings. Make sure your own thoughts are well sorted
- The sense of thought and of concepts is weakened by feeling physically unwell. Because of this it is strengthened by everything which stimulates the life sense of the child
- Keep the life processes of the child in your consciousness
- Ask yourself in the school or parental home: is it worth listening to me?
- Cultivate conversations in your family!

Sense of I
- Remember the root of the sense of I is the sense of touch
- Cultivate perception: pay attention to each other using eye contact, holding hands and through human warmth on a physical, emotional and spiritual level
- Cultivate closeness and reliability instead of distance and fickleness
- Give yourself and your children *time* for meetings!

9. The Competence of Today's Children

It is only healing
When in the mirror of the human soul
The whole community is created
And in the community lives
The power of the single soul.

Rudolf Steiner[50]

At the start of the last century the 'child' became more the centre of focus than ever before in society. In 1900, the Swede, Ellen Kay, declared the twentieth century as the century of the child. In 1907, Rudolf Steiner sowed the seed for the foundations of Waldorf pedagogy with his book *Die Erziehung des Kindes vom Gesichtspunkt der Geisteswissenschaft* — we can see the fruits of this in Waldorf kindergartens and schools throughout the world. Several decades later the Jewish doctor and pedagogue, Janusz Korczak, devised the rights of the child, and with this contributed essentially towards a new human dignity. The organization UNICEF later picked up these children's rights for the children's convention and translated them for our time — a time that has been marked by great changes during the last thirty years. In the seventies A.S. Niell's anti-authoritarian children's movement gave children a new freedom to decide for themselves, but now we are moving back to the other extreme, triggered by the PISA study (Programme for International Student Assessment). This means children's play has been pushed aside in favour of more education again! Politicians are working at increasingly institutionalizing the task of upbringing. Emphasis is placed on looking after children in nurseries and kindergartens so that mothers can work.

Bringing up children is becoming increasingly 'nationalized,' and where institutions have not taken over, computer and television fill the space. At the same time more and more families break up due to the challenges of our times and children are increasingly left to their own devices. Children watch more television at an earlier age, which leads to disturbed and delayed speech development, but also impairment of the entire emotional, cognitive and motor development. These are the consequences, among others, of a decrease in community living. When the media takes over in place of social living together, with its shared tasks and conversations, then inevitably an impoverishment of healthy stimulation and thus also brain networks ensues (see Chapters 7 and 8 about the development of the personality parts and the senses). And all this seen before the background that children have the potential for wide-ranging developmental possibilities!

Old values and traditions hardly play a part in upbringing anymore, and each adult stands alone without being supported by traditional communities. Humankind has reached the absolute

In our time and age the single individual is left completely alone. Old values and traditions do not support us anymore, communities which were the norm in former times are increasingly disbanding

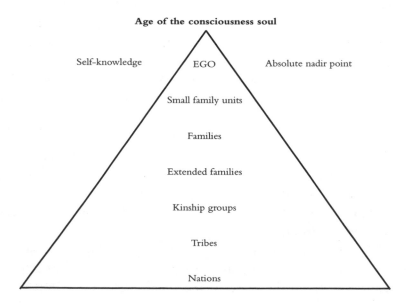

Age of the consciousness soul

Self-knowledge   EGO   Absolute nadir point

Small family units

Families

Extended families

Kinship groups

Tribes

Nations

nadir, and new powers are demanded of us. Our modern time is the age of the consciousness soul, where the greatest challenges have to be faced which demand exactly these qualities of consciousness. The development of the last hundred years is mirrored in our children, up to the point that we speak of a new generation of children: the star children, indigo children, but also of the special ADHD children. Children, and not only those mentioned above, bring different powers with them to the earth, and search for parents and other people to accompany their development. But this works reciprocally, as our children are also developmental helpers for adults. Children come to us with a spectrum of 'knowledge,' which we can also 'learn' from.

Children wish to take part in the development of our I. But how do children experience the I of their parents?

Nowadays parents are mainly engaged with themselves, are nervous, unfocused, have no time and are not really present emotionally. In reality most children experience their parents without the presence of an 'inner conductor' in charge of their emotions, which would enable them to perceive the psyche of the child. This is despite the fact that each child has a deep longing to meet people here on earth where they can develop their sense of I (see Chapter 8), and attain a healthy social I-you relationship.

> Children can act as a mirror which enables us
> to regain our own lost competence, and which
> helps us to discard our unfruitful and unloving
> behavioural patterns. This requires more than just
> democratizing the dialogue between children and
> adults. It means that we have to create a form of
> dialogue which many adults do not manage. *the*
> *personal dialogue of ' equal worth'.*[51]

Children want to co-operate with their parents, particularly if they are talked to as a person and 'equally,' as an equal instead

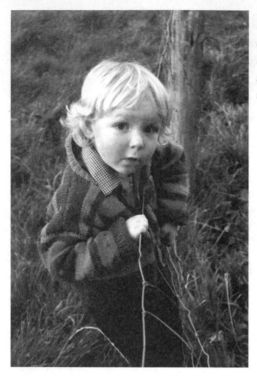

Children mirror our own behaviour with their reactions. In this way, they make us aware of our inappropriate behaviour.

of being reprimanded, put down or treated as if they were not responsible or stupid. Co-operation means that children copy or imitate the adults important to them in their surroundings, that is, 'mirror' their behaviour. A child is also competent when he reacts to his parents' inappropriate behaviour. Children co-operate by unconsciously getting to the bottom of things. They lay their finger on the weak point — on the conflict momentarily disrupting the family.

Aggressiveness as a warning sign

Children lay their finger on the weak point if they feel that their integrity is hurt. Integrity can be hurt at worst by violence, from a slap on the backside to abuse, but also through separation. And even much of what we call upbringing in the normal sense can infringe on the integrity of the child, so that it needs a loophole to escape from the conflict. It does not do this out of opposition, but for self-protection. Jesper Juul has established three theories to explain why children stop co-operating:[52]

- When children 'just do not listen, never mind what we say.' This can usually be put down to the fact that what the parents say is just not worth listening to.
- When children behave destructively and/or antisocially. This always happens if one or several of the adults in their close surroundings also behave like that. It is always the adult who starts! Sometimes consciously, to 'teach the children a lesson,' but usually as the result of their own self-destructive behaviour.
- When children refuse to co-operate. This is either because they have cooperated for far too long despite destructive phenomenon in their family, or because they are subjected to direct assaults on their integrity.

In the following section different examples of the meaning of aggression will be shown. The question is: why does the child or adolescent behave like this? This question is always directed towards the past, to what has happened. With the question: for what reason does the child do this? we look to towards the future.

Aggression creates meetings

Mrs S, the mother of the nine-year-old, Emily, comes to an educational consultation because her daughter, at certain intervals, confronts her aggressively with excessively strong outbursts of anger which she finds difficult to know how to deal with it. Emily is otherwise a quiet girl, who reads a lot and likes being by herself. She has been biting her nails for one year. Emily's mother suspects that her daughter is reacting auto-aggressively, as she separated from Emily's father one and a half years ago. Emily visits her father once a fortnight, sometimes more against her will. Mrs S is a nurse who works weekend shifts during this time. So she is dependant on Emily being looked after well. Emily herself feels insecure in her father's new family where her two older step-siblings live, and does not feel accepted by her father. Mrs S is not able to get in contact with the father.

By letting out her anger against her mother, Emily creates a meeting with her. According to the mother, the arguments are usually thematically connected to the father. But Emily also emerges from her 'shell' during these outbursts of anger and thus creates a meeting with herself. Aggression always has something to do with a strengthening of self-experience and self-confidence.

Mrs S now sees that Emily is mirroring something for her: her own anger against her ex-husband and the fact that she has not got over the separation yet. They are unable to speak together about this theme, and Emily tries to overcome her emotional distress by her outbursts of anger.

Mrs S now sees that she needs to go through a specific grieving process to free Emily from her heavy burden of silence. She also wants to attempt to have a conversation with the father.

Aggression: an open dam

Family B is very loud. Mick is sitting at the computer playing violent games. His mother has already knocked on his door three times and asked him to come for supper. Now she bangs against the door with her fist, because Mick, thirteen years old, locks his door to 'play.' She has no 'power' over him anymore — Mick has been doing what he wants for a long time. He is a head taller than her and is heavily built and his voice has already started breaking. Mick's father is a computer expert and introduced his son to this medium at an early age. He is often away on business trips, and otherwise spends a lot of time at work, leaving the task of upbringing to Mrs B 'At least he used to watch television,' Mrs B says, 'but now he only plays these computer games. Sometimes I don't even know how long he sits in there, because I only get back from the office at 4pm

I think he is addicted to computers! If I set him limits, he threatens me. He's already smashed a glass pane. It's almost impossible to have a conversation with him. There is so much aggression in the room that I often feel helpless and lose my nerve.'

Mrs B feels let down by her husband and challenged to extremes by her son. She can hardly stand the emotional pressure and has problems sleeping at night. She feels her inhibition level is sinking and experiences unpleasant loss of control, where she pounds against the door with her fist, and has even thrown plates at her son.

How is Mick? Mick has removed himself from his family into a world of illusion and games — a world that appears to have helped him to stand the many hours alone as a latchkey child. Mrs B also described her long-standing marriage problems and mentioned that they had never had much of a family life. She always had to work as well to pay off the house. Her son was left to his own devices from an early age.

Mick was increasingly unable to find a sensible outlet for his will-power and emotional energy and instead became frustrated, which led to aggression, either while playing with his computer or physically against his mother.

Mick's integrity had experienced such hurt that 'healing' only seemed possible outside his parental surroundings. For a time he lived on a farm, which gave him access to basic life qualities again. Mick belongs to those adolescents who have to re-learn how to live in 'their house' with their I.

Mrs B managed to start therapy, and separated from her husband during this process. In the meantime Mick lives with his mother again, but has been able to keep up the supporting contact with the farmer.

Mick is a competent adolescent!

From frustration to aggression

It is Sunday evening. I am just returning from a long journey and the last stretch is by regional train. The train is overfull, mainly with teenagers, who are travelling on the special deal weekend ticket. Around me there is unpleasant brawl, several adolescents try to 'out-burp' each other. An elderly lady intervenes: 'You have obviously not learnt to behave yourselves!'

This provocation seems to be successful. One teenager answers: 'Shut up, you old goat!'

The conductor is called, now it gets serious. I feel apprehensive, fear sets in. The teenager quickly becomes violent, feels threatened by the conductor and yet still in the right. His friend intervenes and the adolescent mumbles apologies to the old lady.

It is the last station, the conductor leaves it at that. It could have been worse.

Thoughtful and still a bit caught up by the experience I continue by bus, thinking of my adult children, of garden parties with campfires, of my own adolescence and dealings with alcohol. What was it that made that teenager so aggressive? Was his self-confidence — uninhibited by alcohol — so small, perhaps so hurt, that the old lady could provoke him so?

'Aggression as a warning sign' is the title of this section. The question is: where does the willingness for aggression actually come from?

A normal action turns aggressive when the child feels pushed into a corner, when in a certain sense it looses the connection to reality. This often leads to a lack of consciousness, self-control, and the person concerned becomes self-defensive.

The above examples show that aggressiveness comes from the will, from the actions. The origin of the word 'Aggression' means 'a coming closer,' we can also say: aggression creates a meeting with oneself through the other person because every aggressive clash also leads towards a strengthening of self-experience, of self-confidence.

What is expressed by aggression? To answer this question it helps to differentiate between emotions and actions. What is the difference between anger and aggression? *Anger* is the expression of the emotional, feeling side of a thing, while *aggression* appears as an action, predominantly offensive, and usually destructive.

Aggression can only be understood when I ask about the reason for the action. Why and to what end does the child react aggressively? What triggered it, what lead to the aggressive action? This helps to understand the feelings of the child.

Aggression can occur because of:

- Anger
- Distrust
- Fear
- Stress
- Jealousy
- Hatred
- Boredom ...

In our time and age aggression is aided by several factors. These include lack of excercise, watching television and playing computer games, a premature intellectualization, lack of relationships, heightened competition, negativism in the form of addiction to criticism and a general loss of speech, which means that a conversation and discussion culture cannot be developed.

However, social encounters happen in a community, no matter how small it is! The I can and wants to development itself through the You. This occurs in three big steps. During the first seven years the child gradually brings his I into his will, in the years between seven and fourteen he feels his I stronger in his emotions, and only during puberty does the adolescent experience himself with his I in his thinking. Only then can he have a free and responsible relationship with the community. Our task as parents and educators is to support the child in this process by becoming an *age appropriate* supporter of development.

Speech becomes important for children when they start school. At this point they start conversing together. Previously their meetings have been more physical, now they can name their feelings, even though the child is not yet able to deal with these feelings properly. Only the teenager achieves autonomy in thinking, and can then regulate its feelings. This is the basic condition for being able to handle aggression. Once I have learnt to reflect on a circumstance, an emotion, then I do not need to live out the aggression. The way to achieve this is through the 'centre' of the human being, through the feelings, but also through being felt in the sense of being perceived properly — through the *heart*!

Exercises for self-perception

- According to which values and norms do you act?
- Where do your views and ideas come from?
- Which values represent your real values and which could you perhaps let go?
- How much do the reactions of others affect you if you change your convictions and attitudes?
- How do you appear to other people?
- How do your children/your partner experience you?
- Can you stand up for yourself or would you rather fit in?
- With what can you easily hurt your partner/your children?
- Which behavioural patterns could you easily do without?

Emotional intelligence as the basis for competence

In this section I would like to summarize and extend the above mentioned ideas, looking at them from the viewpoint of 'emotional intelligence.'

The term emotional intelligence describes the ability to correctly perceive emotions, to categorize, regulate and adequately express them. The 'building blocks' of these emotional abilities are already formed during the first years of life, but this process can still be influenced during school age. Emotional abilities are also an essential basis for learning.

The deciding factor is whether the child experiences emotional intelligence in his parents or not. The way in which adults deal with their emotions around the child influences the child from early on.

Example: *Mary has just separated from her partner. Night after night her one-year-old daughter, Lea, wakes up crying. The first few nights Mary takes her into her own bed, which comforts her. After one week Mary has reached her emotional and physical limits. She picks up her daughter in desperation, shakes her and shouts at her, then harshly and coldly puts her back to bed.*

Lea continues screaming for a moment, then she lies in bed quietly with big eyes. Mary cannot get to sleep either: quietly she cries to herself and is tormented by feelings of guilt.

Mary's example shows an extreme situation. If Mary is not able to consciously penetrate the incident, or if this behaviour repeats itself, then emotional messages are conveyed to the child that can have consequences for her whole life. Family life is our first school for emotional education, where we learn how to experience ourselves and how others react to our feelings. Mary has lost her emotional competence as she is under such emotional pressure. To avoid landing in a vicious circle she will probably need outside help. She needs to find a way to regain her energy so that she is able to react to Lea appropriately. Single parents often face exceptional challenges, as they do not have a partner to help them with day-to-day life and support them emotionally in difficult situations. Emotional competence can be practised and mirrored particularly in partnerships.

A further example: *Casper, four and a half, proudly brings his father his afternoon coffee, but at the same time he spills some on the carpet. Quietly he says to himself: 'Doesn't matter, I can mop it up!'*

Casper's father looks up from his newspaper, sees the coffee on the carpet and thunders: 'Goodness, can't you watch out?'

The small boy loses his proud bearing and starts crying. The father does not thank his son, but orders him to go into the kitchen and get a cloth. Will Casper will ever want to bring his father coffee again?'

Casper's father did not empathize with his son, otherwise he would have realized that it is still difficult for a four and a half year old to carry hot coffee. How different it would have been for the son if the father had said: 'Goodness, Casper, you're big enough to bring me my coffee already, but it's still a bit difficult for you. Wait, I'll help you and get a cloth from the kitchen, then we can clean up the carpet together.'

Science repeatedly shows the extensive degree by which children are influenced by whether their parents behave emotionally competently or not.

> Researchers from the university of Washington have found that children from emotionally clever (competent) parents show greater affection for them and have less tension with them compared to those parents who are not able to deal with their feelings. These children are also able to deal with their own feelings better, calm down quicker if there has been an excitement, and are less often flustered. Further the children are psychologically more relaxed, have less stress hormones and other physiological indicators [...] On top of this there are also social advantages: these children are more popular with their peers and teachers consider them to be more socially skilled. According to the judgement of parents and teachers, they have less behavioural problems like roughness or aggressions. Finally, there are also cognitive benefits: these children are more attentive and learn better: The five-year-olds, with the same IQ, whose parents were better emotional teachers, had better marks in grade three in maths and reading; this clearly shows that teaching children emotional abilities prepares them both for school and life. If parents are emotionally skilful, this pays off in a surprising range of advantages for the children across the entire spectrum of emotional intelligence and beyond.'[53]

Emotional intelligence expresses itself, in pre-school children, through capacities which are the basis for learning, in a much more essential sense than already existing knowledge of facts or a premature ability to read. In an article by the *National Center for Clinical Infant Programs* in 1992 seven important characteristics were summarized as the basis for school readiness, I would also like to add, for emotional intelligence:

- *Confidence:* A sense of control and mastery of one's body, behaviour, and world; the child's sense that she is more likely than not to succeed at what she undertakes, and that adults will be helpful;
- *Curiosity:* The sense that finding out about things is positive and leads to pleasure;
- *Intentionality:* The wish and the capacity to have an impact and to act upon that with persistence. This is clearly related to a sense of competence, of being effective;
- *Self-control:* The ability to modulate and control one's own actions in age appropriate ways, a sense of inner control;
- *Relatedness:* The ability to engage with others, based on the sense of being understood by and understanding others;
- *Capacity to communicate:* The wish and the ability to verbally exchange ideas, feelings and concepts with others. This is related to the feeling of trust in others and the joy to get involved with others, including adults;
- *Co-operation:* the ability to balance one's own needs with those of others in a group activity.

Whether children have these capacities when they start school depends mainly on whether parents and educators have helped the child gain a good emotional basis through their own emotional competence.

Parents with emotional competence have developed the following abilities:
- *Know their own feelings.* Many people are not clearly aware of feelings like love, shame or pride and do not know what

these diffuse feelings trigger in them. If I am not able to determine the intensity of my own feelings — then how can I assess how much they affect myself and others?

- *Have empathy.* When we empathize with other people's feelings then they resound within us. This means in relation to children the ability to enter into the feelings of the child, to perceive the intensity of their emotions and the reasons for their behaviour;

- *Learn to deal with their own feelings.* Emotional competence also means knowing when we can reveal our feelings and when it is better to hold them back, to evaluate how the expression or suppression of emotions affects others;

- *Repair emotional damage.* One of the most important abilities in bringing up children is the ability to take on responsibility for the mistakes that we have made. This can mean both asking for forgiveness and making concessions;

- *'Bring everything together.'* This means tuning in to the feelings of those around us and to correctly assess emotional conditions.

Even if you already have children it is not too late to work on your emotional intelligence and create the basis for a competent upbringing.

Exercise questions for creating emotional competence

- Are you intimate with your true feelings? Try to get to know the intensity of your feelings. Writing them down can be helpful. You can classify your feelings from 'weak' to 'strong' to 'overpowering'.

- Perceive the feelings of others. Can you understand why others feel like they do? Can you identify with other peoples life situations and motives?

- Do you have your feelings under control? Can you assess how your feelings affect your children/your partner?

- Can you apologize? Are you able to make concessions? How do you feel when doing so, which feelings and thoughts do you notice in yourself?[54]

10. From Upbringing to Relationship

If a child lives with criticism,
  It learns to condemn.
If a child lives with hostility,
  It learns to fight.
If a child lives with ridicule,
  It learns to be shy.
If a child lives with shame
  It learns to feel guilty.
If a child lives with tolerance,
  It learns to be patient.
If a child lives with encouragement,
  It learns self- confidence.
If a child lives with praise,
  It learns appreciation.
If a child lives with sincerity,
  It learns to be fair.
If a child lives with security,
  It learns to be confident.
If a child lives with appreciation,
  It learns to value itself.
If a child lives with kindness and friendliness,
  It learns to love the world.

                                  After Janusz Korczak

In Chapter 9 it became clear that old values and traditions no longer support us. Children have become competent little personalities, who want us to lead them into life. This means: we must take on this leadership and responsibility. The question is: which qualities do parents and educators need to develop to make this great task succeed?

The above examples have shown how stratified communication is and which levels of personality are involved in it, which often means our I cannot act in freedom, but is quite 'unfree and antiquated.' Suddenly we are touched by high moral ideas, which possibly have less to do with our wish for individuality, but shackle us to old traditions and standards.

Even though I am a 'mother tested by life,' I still feel aggravated when my youngest son slams the door when leaving the room to protest against the list of complaints I have confronted him with, possibly also because I am overstressed. After an occurrence like this I usually have the urge to run after him and say:'What do you think you are doing slamming the door? I forbid you to do that!' Whenever I feel this urge arising within me I see red, because quite obviously doors should not be slammed and I as the mother have the right to...! Here morality speaks paired with parental power, which, if acted out, leads to a dead end situation. The effort then needed to get out of this situation often requires an enormous amount of energy and time. This energy, used sensibly and well thought through, could have prevented the conflict in the first place.

In situations like this I feel moved by the words of the Danish family therapist Jesper Juul, who writes that we need to develop new principles instead of old morals in our dealings with children, leaving our eyes and ears open for the mistakes we inevitably make. We need to be open to these mistakes and take on the responsibility for them, then children can develop in freedom, health and stability. Children help us in this through their competent echoes, which reveal to us where we are stuck in our development. This lets us become conscious of interactions within our families. They primarily reveal the quality of the relationship and only secondarily the quality of upbringing. The deciding factor of how the family feels is the quality of the interactions.

As already mentioned, interactions have a two-fold nature: body language and mimicry, words, attitudes and point of views expressed verbally and at the same time finer nuances, reading 'between the lines:' the underlying attitudes, feelings, conflicts and our whole personal history. In this context Jesper Juul differentiates between *content* and *process*.

The content is *what* we do and say, while the process shows *how* we do and say it. Traditionally we have learnt to believe that content is most important: one does not tell a lie or steal, but

INTERACTION

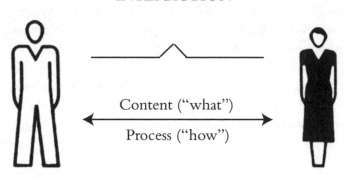

Content ("what")

Process ("how")

At least as important as the message is the way it is expressed. Because depending on how I say it, I express something about my unmentioned feelings and attitudes, my more or less covert conflicts, about my current mood and my relationship to the other person. The communication works without problems if the content and process correspond to each other (from Jesper Juul, Das kompetente Kind, Reinbek 2003, © Rowohlt Verlag, Reinbek *1997).*

sits properly at the table, says 'good day' politely, does not swear, does not talk badly about other people etc.

Interactions occur without problems when content and process correspond with each other — they merge and are of equal importance. This would mean that parents live according to the morals they preach. But often enough the exact opposite is the case.

- Often one hears that parents and children react to a conflict by shouting. If the child becomes louder, the mother often shouts: 'Stop shouting.'
- Family B always talks about daily experiences while eating. Negative experiences are discussed first. The parents are then surprised about the tendency of the children to complain about everything, until it becomes clear to them during counselling that they themselves have started this process by their above-mentioned habit.

- A family of smokers expects its fifteen-year-old son not to smoke, as it is bad for his health. The son does not take his parents seriously, in fact the opposite is true, he uses provocation to show them their inconsistency.

If we, as parents, learn to accept and take seriously what children mirror, then step-by-step we pave the way for us to solve our communication or upbringing problems.

The five basic needs of the human being

Physiological needs

Abraham H. Maslow examined the basic needs of humans in his book *Motivation and Personality*.[55] The needs, which are the basis of the motivational model, are the so called physiological drives. These are basic human needs for food, sleep, bodily contact — safety.

These needs are the strongest of all and can lead, depending on deprivation or fulfilment, to other needs or a different evaluation of individual needs. Somebody who is, for example, lacking food, security, love and respect would probably desire food more than anything else. (Here one could also ask oneself why so many people suffer from obesity). Maslow established that the basic needs have a kind of hierarchical relationship to each other, if the physiological needs are met, then new, higher order needs arise which need to be satisfied.

Safety and security needs

Once the physiological needs have been fairly well satisfied, a new group of needs arise, which Maslow summarizes under the term 'safety and security needs.' These are, for example: security, stability, protection, being free of fear, the need for structure, order, law and limits.

Parents play a central role in this. Rows, physical attacks, separation, divorce or death show particularly strong effects, which can even be physical. Parental fits of rage, threats of punishment and insults can interfere with the children's feeling of security, which then leads to them rejecting their parents — for example, refusing to listen to them — or reacting with obstinacy or tantrums.

Sense of Belonging and love needs

Once the physiological and safety and security needs have been fulfilled, then the need for love, affection, and belonging arises. The absence of parents, partner, friends etc. becomes clearly felt. This need longs for loving relationships with other people, for a place in a group or in the family, which everyone will try hard to attain. The need for love and affection not only means receiving, but also includes giving. love. According to Maslow, the frustration of these needs in our society is the most common cause of disturbances.

Esteem needs

Usually, every person has the need or desire for the highest possible regard by other people. Maslow includes the needs for strength, achievement, ability to manage tasks, competence, trust in the rest of the world, as well as independence and freedom in this need. The satisfaction of the esteem need leads to feelings of self-confidence, strength, the ability and feeling of being useful to the world. The repeated frustration of these needs causes feelings of inferiority, weakness and helplessness.

Significantly, Maslow differentiates between actual competence and achievement, which is based on pure will power, decision and responsibility, from what happens naturally and is easily based on the personal constitution, the own biological destiny. With this he points towards the strengthening of the incarnating I in childhood.

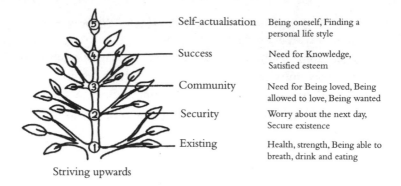

Self-actualisation	Being oneself, Finding a personal life style
Success	Need for Knowledge, Satisfied esteem
Community	Need for Being loved, Being allowed to love, Being wanted
Security	Worry about the next day, Secure existence
Existing	Health, strength, Being able to breath, drink and eating

Striving upwards

The five basic needs of the human being according to Abraham H. Maslow (from Walter Pacher, Ich will doch nur das Beste für mein Kind, © *Verlag Herder, Freiburg im Breisgau, 1st edition 1992).*

Self-actualization needs

Even when all the previously described needs have been satisfied new discontent and disquiet arises if the individual is not able to do what is suited to him. What a human *is able to* be, he *has* to be. The appearance of this need is usually based on the previous satisfaction of the physiological needs as well as the security, love and esteem needs.

Abraham H. Maslow has come to the conclusion that the human being can only be kindly disposed towards his fellow humans beings when the five basic needs are at least partially satisfied. This is true both for children and their parents. The more balanced the needs of family members are, the more harmonious family life can be. If your child reacts with irritation, aggression or rejection then it can be helpful to ask yourself if one of its main needs is not being met. The same is obviously true for partners and parents.

The following exercise can clarify whether individual needs are being met by taking a journey through your house, your garden or the surroundings.

Exercise for the five basic needs of the human being[56]

Imagine you are walking through your (imaginary) house to check out everything. First you go down to the boiler room. You check the temperature and water pressure. You check the oil level, and make sure you will get through the winter. Perhaps you also have a deep freeze and inspect the provisions that you have collected in summer. Now feel lovingly inside yourself: how strongly can you feel your physical reserves? Does your heart beat regularly and strongly, have you got a balanced breathing rhythm? Do you have the necessary reserves for your physical work or do you feel that you are at the end of your tether? This checks your *need for physical survival*.

Now ascend to the first floor, where you check whether all the doors and windows can still open and close. You go to the fuse box and see whether you still have enough fuses left. Perhaps you check the lightning conductor or make sure the gutter is free of leaves. Now feel deeper inside yourself: how secure do you feel in your life situation? Does your family give you support or do you feel like you are a single parent? How secure do you feel at your work place? Do you have the energy and courage to look for new things, or do you withdraw fearfully? This checks on the *need for safety and security*.

Now go into your living room or your own room. Look around it with awareness, let the atmosphere work on you. Do you feel really at home, are you happy with the furnishings, does it allow you to receive guests? Would you be happy if a friend or a colleague came to visit unexpectedly? And now listen within you again: is your need for sociability, for friendship satisfied? Do you like it when people come up to you, or would you rather keep your distance? Do you like opening up and talking to your partner about yourself or are you more careful? This inspection is for your *sense of belonging need*.

And now open the door to your office. Sit down at your desk and go through your letters, is everything in order? How much do you like doing this job, do you keep a housekeeping book, do you have an overview of your money? Do you procrastinate with these tasks or does doing them make you uneasy? Which decisions do you have to make concerning your personal and domestic planning, how much do you like making these decisions or how difficult do you find them?

Listen into yourself again: do you have some people with whom you can share your most innermost feelings and desires, like your partner or a good friend? Do you have the feeling you are valued by your family? Are you successful in your tasks, or do you feel misused by your surroundings? Can you do things like painting, swimming, jogging or something similar that you enjoy, or are you worried about being judged? This inspection is for your *need for success*.

Finally, go out into the garden, look at your house (your life) from a distance. How do you like your home, the inside and the outside? Do you feel good in it, or is it not your style, your idea of comfort? How do you feel in your own skin, how much are you able to lead the life you dream of? Are you at odds with your fate? These questions are for your *need for self-realization*.

Now that you have got to know yourself and your needs in this way and have discovered a bit more about your feeling for your life, perhaps your understanding of conflicts has changed.

Needs have to be taken seriously

We have seen that the more balanced the needs of individual family members are, the more harmonious the family life becomes. Wherever there are tensions in the family one can assume that some basic needs have not been met.

Example: *Libby, the thirteen-year-old daughter of Family K, keeps demanding the attention of the others. She has refused to tidy up her room for weeks. She has already received different sanctions, for example, she is not allowed to bring friends home until she has done her tasks.*

This does not seem to particularly bother Libby. Her parents react with reproach, their upbringing seems to be more authoritarian. Libby is the youngest in the family, she has a sixteen-year-old sister and an eighteen-year-old brother. Seen from the outside one would think that this conflict should be solvable. Referring to the scale of needs it can be helpful to ask questions with regard to Libby's behaviour, as this can lead to a solution of the problem.

The questions could be:
- *In the area of security*: Does Libby feel like an outsider in the family? Is she scared of being dropped completely?
- *In the area of community*: does Libby feel like she is not an equal family member, but rather the 'baby of the family,' and wants to draw attention to herself like this?
- *In the area of self-realization*: Is Libby able to use her own creative will in furnishing her room? Can a new developmentally appropriate step solve the problem with tidying up?

Perhaps the needs of her mother are also not met sufficiently, so that the conflict with Libby becomes so important and difficult to solve. Because of this it can be sensible to ask oneself as parents how much one's own needs are met. The more satisfied my basic needs are, the more I am able to be a good mother and wife or a good father and husband.

It is only with the heart that one can see rightly! To really be able to hear with the heart, I need to become conscious of myself and listen towards the heart of the other, my child, with this liberated energy. I need to learn to ask questions which others can hear, because then they feel seen and touched inside by me.

In this way we can learn to recognize, understand and differentiate conflicts. We can learn whether a conflict is of basic needs, or of values. The step we have to make is listening, both to the one's own internal feelings and also towards the child. Only through unconditional listening can we find out about each other.

About the art of listening

We can distinguish between four basic techniques of listening:

• *Passive listening*

Passive listening works as a definite non-verbal message, which signals to the child that it can speak:

— I would like you to say what you feel.

— I accept your feelings.

— I leave the decision up to you as to what you would like to tell me.

Passive listening encourages children to speak about their feelings. In this way one often reaches the deeper lying problems. But when children talk about their problems, they usually expect more than just silent listening!

• *Attentive listening*

Passive silence avoids the notorious 'communication blocks,' which so often convey to the child that its messages are not acceptable. On the other hand it is not proof that we are really listening, giving it attention. Because of this it is helpful to show that one is following internally by making appropriate gestures and giving verbal support. This can be, for example, an interjection like ' I understand' or nodding your head etc. this transmits the feeling that one is interested and that the speaker's statements have been accepted.

• *'Door openers' or 'invitations'*

Sometimes children need additional support during conversations to be able to talk about their feelings or problems. Such 'invitations' can be:

'Would you like to talk about it?'

'I would be interested to know what you think about that.'

The questions should be open and unbiased, and give the child the chance to speak about further aspects of the problem.

• *Active listening*

Here the listener does not convey a message, he solely mirrors the directly preceding message of the child by giving corresponding echoes. To do this he repeats the message in his own words. Through this echo he shows actively that he understands the spoken words both acoustically and their meaning.

Examples

• Child: 'I am just too stupid to understand the maths problem!'
Mother/Father: 'You mean you are not clever enough and you can't understand it?'
Child: 'Yes, exactly:'

• Child: 'They are always so unfair to me at school:'
Mother/father: 'You feel unfairly treated by the others, that makes you feel upset:'
Child: 'Yes, then I feel so alone in the class.'

• Child: 'I don't want to go to my childminder.'
Mother/father: 'So you don't like going to Marion when I have to go to work.'
Child: 'No, not at all. I don't want to go. I miss you then.'
Mother/father: 'You would like me to be here for you in the morning. Is there anything that can help make it less difficult for you?'
Child (ponders): Maybe if I had your coat, it always smells like you.'

Now a counter-example for active listening:

• Child: 'I wish we still lived in Ammers.'
Mother/father: 'Why do you think that?'
Child: 'I haven't got any new friends here, nobody to play with.'
Mother/father: 'Well, I bet there are some nice boys in your class who would like to play with you.'
Child: 'But why does nobody ask me then?'

Mother/father: 'Perhaps you need to ask and shouldn't be so shy.
You should just dare for a change!'
Child (withdraws): 'You don't understand me at all.'

I am sure that the mother or father here wanted to help in the
best sense, but it still went wrong. The problem of the child is
not dealt with with real understanding. The parent immediately
make a counter-statement. When the boy is not able to agree
with this the parents express an evaluation — the focus of the
problem is shifted and it almost seems as if the parents think it
is the boy's own fault if he does not find any friends. His real
feelings were not touched upon and so his attitude towards the
problem could not be changed.

One can learn active listening, but one also has to practise
it, similar to learning to play an instrument, which also needs
continuous practice to achieve results.

Most people initially feel that active listening is disconcert-
ing and unnatural. It should not become 'parrot like,' where you
repeat exactly what the other says. Rather relate to the feelings
of the child with your own words. This will help the child feel
understood and enable it to open up more unconditionally.

Active listening in the family means:
• Strong feelings can lessen as they have been expressed;
• Feelings become friendlier;
• Listening helps develop greater trust between the members;
• Children show more responsibility;
• You can learn to trust your child;
• You will be able to accept more;
• It makes you happy to help;
• The child becomes an independent individual.

Some tips and guidelines for active listening:
• Accept that active listening will seem unnatural to you at the
  start;
• You can only control active listening if you practise it sufficiently;

- Do not give up too quickly;
- You will never know the abilities of your children if you do not give them the chance to solve their problems themselves;
- Find out when active listening is not appropriate (are your personal problems too central at the moment? Have you not got any time at the moment?);
- Try to use the other techniques of listening: passive listening, attentive listening and 'door openers.' You do not have to repeat everything your child says;
- Use active listening when strong emotions are concerned and when your child is dependent on being accepted.
- Only give your children advice when they need it.

Educating towards conflict ability

Active listening; from you-messages to I-messages

When I 'listen actively' (see Chapter 10) I try and understand the message and problems of others, if possible so succinctly that they see their situation more clearly because of my contribution. The most essential part of active listening is to remain completely connected to the other person, to his needs. If this succeeds, then he will feel understood and motivated to contribute something towards solving the conflict.

Correct active listening does not accuse the speaker and because of this what is said can be accepted. In general it is always important to avoid accusations in conversations as much as possible. I-messages are one way of talking to other people so they do not feel attacked, while you-messages always have an underlying accusation.

I try and explain my needs and problems with an I-message. This means the listener can understand me in the correct way. Instead of the reproach which always sounds through a you-message ('You always do …'), an I-message expresses how it makes me feel when the other person does something that annoys me. The most important part of the I-message is that I remember to talk only about myself and my needs, without rebuking or giving small side-sweeps. If this succeeds, then the other person can take me seriously and listen to my arguments. A correct I-message, which is free from reproach, does not put unnecessary obstacles in the path of the other person's understanding.

Unfortunately, it is initially easier to express oneself in you-messages, as this requires less self-reflection. Without further ado the responsibility for ones own emotions are transferred onto the other person. In this way the spoken words cannot reach their goal — you-messages usually lead to resistance and obstinacy. The following is also true for you-messages:

- They cause destructive arguments and accusations of one another;
- They make children feel guilty, put down, criticized and hurt;
- They cause children to seek revenge on their parents and the wish to put them down;
- They convey a lack of respect for the needs of the other person.

  'You are annoying me:'

  'Do you have to always get so dirty?'

  'You go to your room now!'

  'You do what I say!'

  'I couldn't sleep because of you.'

  'You don't have to shout so loudly.'

I am sure that everybody is familiar with these or similar messages from their own childhood, and what the reactions are. Children become obstinate and refuse to change. You-messages harm the self-respect of the child. It is no wonder that they take revenge by using you-messages themselves, which then end with hurt feelings, tears, slammed doors and threats of punishment.

Let us go back to Libby:

Mother: 'Right, Libby, I want your room to be clean and tidy in one week!'

Libby: 'I don't think so, it's my room and I'll do what I want with it!'

Mother: 'You don't have to help with the household duties at all, so the least you should be able to do is keep your room tidy, but you can't even manage that!'

Libby: 'If I wanted to, I could do it, but I don't want to. And that's it!'

Mother: 'I don't understand you, you are making life difficult for us all with this continuous struggle.'

Libby: 'Huh, I don't care!' (She leaves the kitchen slamming the door).

Libby's mother has made all the classical you-messages mistakes. She has pushed Libby into a corner, and has even made her feel responsible for the well-being of the family.

How the conflict could have proceeded differently is shown by the new attempt of the mother after several counselling sessions:

Mother: 'I think it's important to talk to you about your room again.'

Libby: 'But I don't!'

Mother: 'I guess you've had enough of this theme, is that right?'

Libby: 'Yes, exactly!'

Mother: 'I have thought about the conflict with the room and have come to the conclusion that I made a mistake.'

Libby (pauses, looks at mother): 'Yes, that could be.'

Mother: 'I notice I find it very difficult to deal with mess. I feel depressed when I know that one of the rooms in the house looks like that and I have no influence on it.'

Libby (already in a milder mood): 'Actually I know that. I don't feel too good in my room any more either, but when you all attack me, I don't want to do anything anymore.'

Mother: 'So you would actually like to do something about your room?'

Libby: 'Yes, but not just tidy it up. I would also like to make it a bit cooler.'

Mother: 'Is there anything I can help you with?'

Libby (hesitantly, then more open): 'To be honest, I think it would be great if you could help me sort things out because I have so many childhood things in my room I don't need anymore. But I don't know by myself what can be put away. I am still attached to everything and I can't decide.'

Mother: 'I'll do that gladly, Libby. But I need a day for it where I have enough time. Unfortunately that's Tuesday, your riding day.'

Libby: 'Okay, I'll see to it that I can miss riding. This is important to me. Thanks, mum.'

By listening actively and talking about herself, Libby's mother took over the responsibility for the situation again. Thomas Gordon calls I-messages 'responsibility messages' for the following reasons:

- An adult who sends an I-message takes on the responsibility for his own inner condition (he listens into himself to see what he can hear) and he shows his responsibility by conveying this self-evaluation openly to the child;
- I-messages leave the responsibility to change unacceptable behaviour to the child. It does not feel forced by the adult to do something against his will. At the same time I-messages avoid negative judgements and strengthen the will of the child towards consideration and helpfulness.[57]

I-messages fulfil three important criteria for a 'promising' communication:
1. They are they are the most likely messages to further willingness to change;
2. They do not contain much negative evaluation of the child;
3. They do not harm the relationship.

A good I-message does not infer things like: 'You should do this or that.' Rather they enable children and adolescents to develop their own solutions together with adults for their problems. These solutions are often surprisingly creative and would perhaps never have occurred to adults. Children want to find their own solutions because they do not like to see their needs refused.

I had the chance to observe this beautifully a few years ago with a stubborn conflict I had with my then ten-year-old son. He desperately wanted to let his hair grow, but I only discovered this after some time. Up until this point we had led quite a few discussions about hair cutting. I just repeatedly admonished that his hair was too long and hung in his face. With which he shrugged his shoulders and said: 'But I don't want to go to the hairdressers.'

One day I sat down with him and said. 'We have talked about cutting your hair so often now and I can't force you to go to the hairdresser. I am now dependant on your help, what we can do together. Do you have an idea?' with which my son answered: 'Yes, I want to talk to Hans.' (Hans is his twenty-year-old brother).

'Why with Hans?'

'Because Hans can tell me how he managed to grow his ponytail without his hair hanging in his face.'

After this talk the problem was not a problem anymore, because I had discovered something about the intentions of my son, which he had withheld from me because of my demands.

All these aids mentioned above lead to 'promising' communication. Paying attention to the needs of the participants, active listening, using I-messages — they all have something to do with attentiveness, patience, tolerance and acceptance towards the stranger. They help to achieve educational goals without using power, and assist children in their development of their competence, especially their social competence. This way of dealing with conflicts is an up-to-date reaction towards the increasing self-confidence of children during the last thirty years.

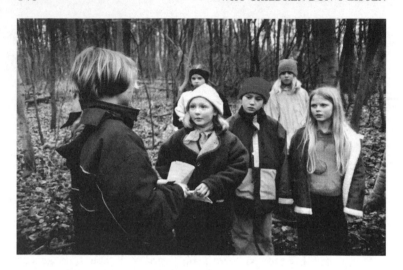

If our upbringing is not based on power and authority, but on attentiveness, patience and tolerance, when we speak to children and adolescents as an "equal" partner, without giving them responsibility which they cannot yet carry, then this helps them to develop social competence.

If we as parents learn to say goodbye to our old behavioural patterns of moralizing, informing, warning and judging, then upbringing becomes the basis for a healthier relationship with the child. If we stop making our children responsible for large parts of our behaviour, by sending encoded messages, and instead say with I-messages what is really happening, then our children will be able to develop new social abilities.

If children don't have to hear: 'You are driving me mad!,' or 'Do you always have to be so loud?' but rather perhaps: 'I am tired, I have a headache when the piano is so loud — can you please play a bit quieter?' then it becomes a criticism of the thing and not the person, and the other person does not need to feel attacked. When you work with the techniques of active listening and I-messages you will soon notice that tensions in the family decrease. As children learn by the example of their parents and mirror their behaviour, the reactions you receive from them will also change and become more positive.

Once you have learnt to listen actively and articulate I-messages then you have cast away an old part of yourself. Possibly you will also experience this as a loss, an uncertainty, an inner 'nakedness.' The old authoritarian ideas do not support us anymore. In their stead a new quality will develop in your relationship with your child, which is influenced by closeness, respect and 'equality.' Only once I have understood the logic of the child, and when he or she has found the willingness to speak about his or her problems and needs openly, freely and without fear, is it possible for me do without power in upbringing.

This can be summarized in two essential basic requirements:

- I have to understand the inner need of the child;
- The child has to sense that I understand him or her.

Exercises for sending I-messages

Imagine you are in the situations described below, relate to the you-messages and then write your I-message in the third column.

At the end of the table you will find suggestions for solving these conflicts based on I-messages.

Situation	You-message	I-message
1. The mother is phoning, while the three-year-old child is emptying the sewing box and unwinding the thread.	'You are messing everything up, you silly little thing:'	

2. The child is near-
ing a socket with
a screwdriver and
wants to drill in it.

The mother seizes it:
'You obviously want
to get an electric
shock!'

3. The thirteen-year-
old daughter comes
home by bus one
and a half hours late.
The mother is stand-
ing waiting at the
bus stop.

'Obviously you think
imagine you can do
anything. You must be
out of your mind to
make me so worried.'

4. The pubescent
son turns his CD
player up full blast so
that the bass drones
through the house.

'Can't you be more
considerate towards
other people?!'

5. The parents want
to go to the theatre
in the evening, a
babysitter is com-
ing to help out.
You have arranged
with your three
children (eight, five
and three) that they
have to be ready for
bed by the time the
babysitter comes.
Instead the chil-
dren are fighting,
the youngest one is
grasping his moth-
er's leg and crying.

'It's so mean that
you are not sticking
to the agreement.
You are spoiling our
whole visit to the
theatre.' (You-mes-
sages in the plural!)

6. The children come
home from school
and complain that
lunch is not ready.
The mother had
imagined that they
would help. Instead
they sit down at the
piano and on the
easy chair.

'You're so badly-
behaved! P., you
are an absolute lazy
bones, and you, K.,
also only wait to be
served!'

7. The mother has
just cleaned the
house when her
child comes in with
dirty shoes.

'You really are a
dirty person, you are
making everything
dirty again!'

8. The daughter
keeps using her dad's
razor to shave her
legs.

'Do you always have
to use my razor, all
your hair's still stick-
ing to it.'

9. The mother is
vacuuming the car-
pet. The child keeps
pulling the plug out
of the socket.

'You are naughty!'

10. The child has
been noticeably
quiet the whole
day. She seems to
be dejected, but the
mother does not
know why.

'Now come on, stop
grumping. Either
your mood improves
or you can go to
your room. You don't
have to take every-
thing so seriously.'

Suggestions for I-messages for the situations 1–10:

1. 'I can't telephone properly because I am worried my sewing things will get mixed up.'
2. 'I am scared you will get an electric shock, that is why I don't want you to play with it.'
3. 'I was worried about you and am also annoyed that I didn't hear anything from you, what happened?'
4. 'I know you like having loud music at the moment, but I can't stand it because I can only hear the bass, and it's going right through me.'
5. Father: 'I am annoyed that you are not sticking to our agreement. I think it is a shame that your mother and I can't look forward to the theatre properly because we have to shout at you.'
6. 'I'm disappointed that neither of you feel the need to help me. And I have the impression that you expect me to have the meal ready on the table for you. So I feel like your waitress.'
7. 'Stop, I've just cleaned, and then I'm particularly sensitive if you come in with dirty shoes. Please take them off.'
8. 'I don't like it when you use my razor for your legs. I find it disagreeable having bits of your hair in my face.'
9. 'I'm terribly rushed, and it really makes me angry if I'm held back by having to put the plug back into the socket. I don't feel like playing when I have to work.'
10. 'I am sorry to see you so unhappy, but I don't know how to help you because I don't know why you are upset.

11. Family Conflict Management

The term 'conflict management' shows that a family is also a kind of business which needs guide and support to managed conflicts sensibly. Families are businesses which need a lot of 'servicing,' but unfortunately neither society nor the people concerned are sufficiently aware of this. So how can they acquire the appropriate esteem? Conflict management in a company, school and the work force in general is accepted by society, and conferences and supervision are offered to them. It is only in the family, the primordial cell of society where the roots of later social ability are formed, where parents and children are expected to cope without help. Overcoming this point of view is the most difficult step. Before mothers or fathers register for parental courses they usually struggle for far too long with the question: 'Why can't I do this alone? My parents managed it!'

In the previous section several techniques were described which can help steer and finally solve existing conflicts in day-to-day situations. A further point, which has a harmonizing effect on living together, is the family conference.

The family conference

In most family relationships problems and questions are 'swept under the carpet' and are not dealt with due to lack of time and also contact. To change this it is useful to arrange a family meeting at regular intervals, where all the family members take part and can discuss the things concerning them in the family.

Let us take a look at the family of five, Family K, which consists of mother, father, seven-year-old daughter, Ella, nine-year-old son, Tom, and thirteen-year-old daughter, Lena. The usually weekly family conference is a firm part of Family K's life. The reason for starting this was conflict with Lena four years ago. Mrs K felt completely overwhelmed by the personality changes which took place in her daughter when she was nine years old. Lena started to shake the foundations of all the family habits. She started looking towards her friends and their home life and hardly ever held back her criticism. Family K decided to start a family meeting every Sunday evening.

Mr and Mrs K talked about the form and content of this 'meeting' in advance. They felt it was important not to use this meeting as an educational measure, but that it should serve as an organ of perception for their family life. They planned in an hour for their first meeting, where they could be completely undisturbed by others. This meant, for example, not answering the telephone and directing their attention solely towards the family group.

The parents started the family conference with the theme: 'What I have been wanting to say for a long time!'

Mrs K: 'I am pleased that we have managed to start this regular family meeting today. I would like everybody to be able to say what concerns them, but also to express the good points. If someone has an idea about what to change in the family, then I would be interested in hearing it.'

Lena: 'I think it's great that we are sitting here together, in school we also sometimes talk to our teachers about these things. — I want to say something today about going to bed.'

Tom: 'I don't really want to share a room with Ella anymore.'

Ella: 'I can sleep on my own now!'

Mr K: 'I also have a wish, but first I suggest that mother or I write down all the points we want to discuss and then we can decide when everybody can have a turn.'

Tom: 'Can't we throw a dice? I just got a new coloured dice, everybody can have a colour.'

Ella: 'Yes, I want to be red.'

Tom's suggestion was gladly taken up, it was a nice idea and in this playful way the younger children are integrated better.

Mr K: 'Now I'd still like to express my concern. I look forward to seeing you when I come home in the evening, and also like hearing what you have done all day. You always have a lot to tell me (his eyes are resting on the children). When I'm listening to your mum and you also want to tell me something, then I notice how difficult it is for you to let me speak to her. Sometimes I get quite angry and notice that I don't really feel like listening to you. So I would like us to think about what we could do, perhaps you have an idea.'

Mrs K: 'I've just got this book which is going to become our 'meeting book.' Dad's wish is already in here; Your dad will now add your matters of concern. Now I want to tell you my point: I'd like to have a cleaning day once a week, where everybody takes on some of the housework. It's difficult for me to manage all the work by myself. I have written a list of all the things that need to be done throughout the week. I'd like to go through it with you and then we can decide who wants to do what.'

Ella: 'But I also want to do something!'

I think we can now let Family K finish discussing their points and join them again at the end of their family meeting ...

Family K was successfully able to solve all their concerns together, as the parents did not send any you-messages nor use their authority. They were able to appeal to the competence of their children:

- Ella is now allowed to sleep by herself, which she is very proud of;
- Tom is allowed to renovate the small washroom with his father and can look forward to his own small room;
- Lena is allowed to stay up for another three quarters of an hour. But they agreed to see for a while how she feels in the morning;
- Mrs K. was surprised how many offers of help she received. Everyone was happy to take on something,
- Mr K arranged with all three children that they leave him and their mother alone to talk in the sitting room for fifteen minutes every day. During this time the older children will look after Ella;

At the end of the family meeting they arrange to sit down together again a week later to see how the new agreements have worked out. During the week they hang a piece of paper onto the pin board where everyone can write down or draw what they would like to discuss in the following family meeting.

If it is not so easy to solve

One can use a classic six-point resolution procedure to help find solutions in the family meeting.[58] This procedure has worked well for business and industry, so why not for families, particularly if the family cannot come to an agreement during the family meeting. In this case it is almost essential to have a structure to avoid getting caught up in discussions.

These are the six points:
1. Make notes of the needs and identify and define the problem;
2. Collect suggested solutions without valuing them (brainstorming);
3. Evaluate the suggested solution and set the goal;
4. Choose a solution;
5. Plan and implement the solution;
6. Check the result.

Here is an example from my own family: in our family slamming doors, particularly in relation to anger, is a recurrent theme, mainly because of our thirteen-year-old, second youngest child. Certain examples, that is, experiences with older siblings and occasionally me as the mother, had certainly paved the way for this problem. As one day we had reached the limit of endurance my husband and I decided to discuss slamming doors at the family conference:

1. We described how door-slamming affected us, how everyone gets a fright, how we have to think of the other family

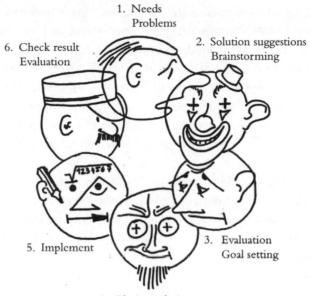

1. Needs
   Problems

6. Check result
   Evaluation

2. Solution suggestions
   Brainstorming

5. Implement

3. Evaluation
   Goal setting

4. Choose solution

Six point resolution procedure (from Walter Pacher, Ich will doch nur das Beste für mein Kind. © Verlag Herder, Freiburg im Breisgau, 1st edition 1992).

in our semidetached house, and apart from that how we also become angry about it. This clarified the fact that we as parents do not want to live like that. Naturally counter-arguments followed like: 'But when I'm angry I want to slam doors!'

2. Although we could not find an agreement we looked for possible solutions together. The suggestions ranged from shutting one's ears to saying sorry, from unscrewing the door handle to paying a 'fine.'

3. We then went through all the possibilities from the point of view of which one could act as a deterrent, so that nobody would want to slam doors, and how that would affect everybody.

4. We decided to get a family piggy bank for everybody to pay a euro each time they slammed a door. There was

more tension during the discussion about how much the fine should be, but this could be eliminated by having a goal for the collected money.

5. Now we still had to decide who was going to get the piggy bank, where it should stand, when we should empty it and what we should do with the money. The suggestion came to donate it to a good cause, but not everyone could accept this proposal. Finally we agreed to go out for a meal with the money so that everybody profited from it.

6. The result could be seen quickly as immediately door slamming happened noticeably less. I myself had to pay in a first euro fairly soon, though the anger already subsided when I shouted into the dining room while slamming the door: 'A euro, I know!'

This shows that some 'rules' or basic techniques of communication can play a deciding part in the success of the conversations. We have got to know them all in the preceding chapters:

- Make time for conversations with the family.
- Look the children in the eyes when you are talking to them. Only then do they feel talked to inside.
- Use the technique of active listening (see Chapter 10).
- Use I-messages (see Chapter 10).
- Make sure that you are 'completely there' and not distracted.
- Approach the problems discussed with a questioning attitude. Why is my child discontented with something? Where do the suggested changes lead?
- Think of your 'inner team,' of the different impulses which live in your wishes and ideas. Clarify for yourself which member of your inner team is speaking out of yourself at the moment (see Chapter 12).

All these building blocks can make the family conference into a valuable part of your family life. Remember that you as the adult carry the responsibility for the interactions in your family. Children cannot do this yet, because they are still

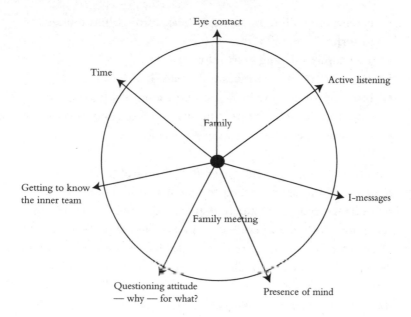

developing physically and emotionally. They want and have to practise their behaviour on us. A family meeting is a good opportunity for all participants to work at their respective 'tasks' in communication.

Children feel taken seriously at the family meeting. Stubborn children can suddenly become interested conversation partners who are willing to compromise. The family meeting, used properly, has a very reconciliatory, satisfying, and connecting effect on the entire social organism of the family. In this way children learn the ability to deal with conflict in later life!

A family meeting can succeed when:
- It is not used as a tool for upbringing;
- The parents do not use their power;
- Everybody practises the different forms of listening;
- I-messages, not you-messages, are sent;
- Parents take on the responsibility for its progress;
- Parents want to get to know their inner team;

- Parents are willing to see and break through old transaction patterns;
- The family meeting is structured;
- There are no disturbances from outside;
- Problem solving methods are known and integrated;
- The interval until the next family meeting is not too long;
- Previous agreements are kept to reliably.

Family meetings like this contribute towards a deepening of humanity. Courage is needed to take part in the different levels, to overturn old rules and find new, individual limits. When I reveal myself to other people, to a partner and child, by daring to place myself in the midst of day-to-day happenings, then I show myself as the person I really am. You-messages still veil something of myself, perhaps my 'shadow' or my 'double.' I-messages show that I am a person who can be hurt or embarrassed, fearful, disappointed, angry or discouraged. Revealing how I feel means I am 'seen' by others. What do other people think of me?

Perhaps each person knows the fear of being recognized. Do we have to hide this fear from everyone? Or is the family perhaps the place where human beings with all their strengths and weaknesses are allowed to be themselves?

> When parents and children learn to be open and
> honest with each other, then they are no longer
> 'strangers in the same house.' Parents can enjoy
> being the parents of a real person — and the chil-
> dren are blessed with real people as parents.[59]

12. Self-discipline as the Basis of Bringing up Children

Getting to know your inner team

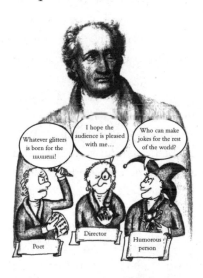

Three "souls in the breast" of the Faust author, derived from the "prelude in the theatre" (from Friedemann Schulz von Thun, Miteinander reden, *Volume 3, Reinbek 2005, © Friedemann Schulz von Thun).*

Goethe spoke of the 'two souls' residing within the breast. In the prelude to *Faust* he even had 'three souls within the breast' on the stage. We can see the poet projects his inner conflicts onto the outer stage, giving them a name and letting them talk and argue together. In this case the art of poetry allows such creative steps.

I would also like talk about art in relation to our theme: *social art*. Heinz Zimmermann describes conversation as a pre-stage to a future social art; an art which forms human relationships as an

'art of the time.' This works creatively through the medium of
I-perceptions of others and oneself in relation to a recognized
higher human image.[60]

Friedemann Schulz von Thun has contributed valuably
to this theme with his research in communication. He created an 'inner stage' for the different souls in the breast of
the person, enabling him, in the sense of an 'inner dynamic
group,' to develop clarity, order and new energy. This allows
him to develop some distance from the day-to-day person in
himself. Schulz von Thun calls these stage actors the 'inner
team.' They constitute the different voices or personality
parts in a person.

Each member of the inner team has a message and a name
related to this message (see below). As a rule the messages are
based on our experiences, on things that have happened during
our life which have left an impression (see also Chapter 7).

Each inner team has a team leader, a director on the inner
stage. He has a difficult task as it can become quite turbulent
on this stage.

Try to get to know the actors on your inner stage. Which
impulses do their actions convey? Perhaps you have a person inside you who is always in a hurry or too hasty. Or do
you have someone in your inner team who immediately
becomes suspicious? Or someone who does not like to be
noticed, who is quickly embarrassed? Give all these inner
actors names, as this often makes it easier to establish a more
'personal' contact.

Members of the inner team can be:
- The hurried one
- The suspicious one
- The shy one
- The single-minded one
- The bundle of nerves
- The adapted one
- The hard-hearted one

- The one in command
- The embarrassed one

... and many more actors, depending on personality.

Exercise examples

- Your thirteen-year-old daughter is caught stealing eye-shadow. The police are called; and they bring your daughter home in a police car. You live in a housing estate where everyone sees everything. What do your inner team members say?
- You are in the supermarket with your two-year-old child. At the checkout she wants to have the nice and colourful sweeties in a bottle, which you do not want her to have. Your child arches her back and starts screaming. How does your inner team react?
- Your nine-year-old son comes home from school covered in blood and crying, he was beaten up on the way home by older boys. You know your son is a shy boy. What does your inner team say?
- Your husband/wife comes home in the evening. You have had an exhausting day with the children, visits at the doctor, the children's music lessons, etc. the housework has suffered somewhat under these circumstances. You see dissatisfaction and annoyance on your partner's face, he/she bangs the doors loudly, and on the whole seems irritated. Do you relate this non-verbal expression to yourself? Let your inner stage actors start a discussion about this theme.

Sometimes the discussions of the inner team-mates go on endlessly, and possibly fruitlessly, if the director or team leader does not intervene and start a team meeting where the inner conflicts can be worked through. Here I would like to introduce you to the five phases of inner conflict management according to Friedemann Schultz von Thun:[61]

Five phases of inner conflict management

1. Identification of the participants
Who is involved in the conflict? Which members of your inner team have formed an alliance? Reserve a chair or cushion for each participant in the conflict.

2. Self-revelation of the antagonists
What does each antagonist have to say, what do they stand for? Which feelings do you have while they are talking? Here it can be helpful to take on the role of the antagonist by sitting on the respective chair or cushion.

3. Dialogue: discussing and arguing together
Discuss a conflict between the participants, speaking to the relative antagonist. It can be helpful for you sit on the respective chairs/cushions when taking on the roles of the different participants. Discuss the 'true' feelings (bitterness or mutual contempt).

4. Reconciliation and partial acceptance
Why is good about the antagonist? What can I learn to value in him? How do we depend on each other so that our whole person can live well?

5. Team creation and decision-making by the team leader or director
The director of the inner stage, who is leading the inner team meeting, decides from a higher point of view: Who should have precedence in which situation? How can they mutually complement each other? Who should be allowed to take up more space in the future, who needs to remain in the background?

This five-phase programme is meant as an aid to self-help. In acute or very complicated cases it does not replace professional counselling. It is well suited as a partner exercise, but also in parental groups as an autodidactic supervision. It is also an excellent tool for people who want to work at their personality development by themselves.[62]

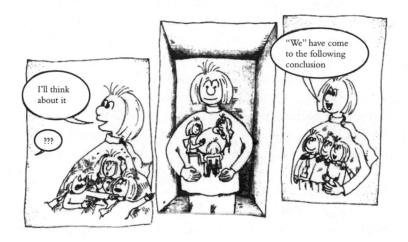

Summoning an "inner meeting" (from Friedemann Schulz von Thun, Miteinander reden, Volume 3, Reinbek 2005, © Friedemann Schulz von Thun).

Soul hygiene as the basis for a new perception

'Soul hygiene' is probably an unusual term for many of you. Despite this I would like to use it here, and also with regard to hygiene in general. Hygiene is the teaching of health and its maintenance. We can differentiate between environmental, social and emotional hygiene. The latter is aimed at the optimal adjustment of the individual to his social and civilization environment, and thus towards a preservation of the health of his emotions and intellect. Environmental hygiene examines the relationship between health and outer life circumstances (water, ground, air, food, clothing and work). Social hygiene is concerned with the effect of societal interconnections on the health of individuals and collectives.

Rudolf Steiner has given self-discipline instructions in many of his lectures. The person employing them can strengthen his life-energy, his soul and his I. These exercises help with presence of mind and stability in life and soul, which in turn creates a healthier sense of relationships and contributes towards the physical health of the human being. The five basic needs of the human being according to Maslow (see Chapter 10) can become more conscious in this way.

Mothers and fathers have to be able to withstand high pressure without many breaks in day-to-day life. This often leads to impatience, feeling rushed and feelings of unfairness. Making a time of peace and inner calm despite all the things that need to be done regenerates, strengthens and contributes towards the presence of mind necessary, but is so difficult to achieve particularly in our fast moving time.

You only need a few minutes a day for the following exercises. Rudolf Steiner recommends not to start with all the exercises at the same time, but to devote oneself to the first exercise for a period of about a month, then to add the second one while keeping up the first one, after four weeks to add the third one and so on, until you can employ all six exercises beside each other. You will notice that with sufficient creativity in the moments of exercise habits develop which you will not want to miss later, as they stand like a spiritual support in the soul. The enables you to shape your life more effectively and consciously using your I.

Subsidiary exercises of Rudolf Steiner[63]

Controlled thought

This first exercise is for looking at the process of thought. Particularly in day-to-day life with children we experience such a host of impressions and actions that our thinking becomes chaotic and associative. Anxiety is often the result.

Try to concentrate on a particular object for about five

minutes a day, if possible without deviating from the subject. A simple object is the most suitable.

Once you have experienced how useful it is for achieving inner calmness and concentration to occupy oneself in thoughts of a pin or a matchstick for just a few minutes you will know the value of this exercise. You can ask inner questions to the object like: What parts belong to the object, what do they consist of, how are they put together, what is its design? Who invented it and why? What was the past history of the object etc. You will be able to come up with your own questions. It is only important that the questions have something to do directly with the chosen object.

You can either change the object daily, or keep one object to think about every day over a longer period of time. In the latter case new interest and energy in the object has to be developed more strongly every day. This exercise is useful for every day as it teaches us to perceive the process of thought. Rudolf Steiner also recommends that we think logically about the matter when we hear illogical thoughts.

Will initiative
This exercise trains the power of the soul over the will. Think of any action without a specific purpose which you would like to do at a certain time. Plan, for example, to put your right finger to your nose or to stroke through your hair in the morning at 9.45am. It can be a completely banal action deliberately, so you need a strong will to do it.

If you missed the time, which initially happens repeatedly as we humans live strongly in our habits, then just determine a new time. You can gradually add more actions of this kind throughout the day, but sometimes less is more!

You will notice that this kind of action strengthens the will and works against the dissatisfaction and restlessness of our time. In day-to-day life this exercise can help to strengthen the logical consistency of one's own actions (and speaking is also an action!) and to increasingly overcome inconstancy and disharmony.

Equanimity

The goal of this exercise is to develop a greater stability in the face of fluctuating feelings such as desire and suffering, joy and pain. The alternation between being up one minute and down the next should be transformed into a serene mood, a kind of inner calmness. This exercise builds nicely on what we have seen in the previous chapters, as it is helpful to familiarize yourself with your feelings and gestures before starting this exercise.

Resolve to pay attention to your feelings in day-to-day life, and then transform them as soon as they arise. If, for example, you have a tendency to start shouting whenever you are angry, then the task can be to perceive the anger, but to moderate or refrain from acting out the action, the shouting. The exercise can also mean that someone who has difficulties showing feelings of joy tries to show them better. It is helpful to look back at the practised exercise once a day, perhaps also to write the experiences down in a book, this makes one become even more responsible for the actions.

> The goal of this exercise is to develop a rich, free and as impartial as possible life of feelings and at the same time to have complete power over its ups and downs, this means to be centred in oneself, creating a space were sympathy and antipathy are weighed up against each other and in which feelings can then emerge most intensely.[64]

Positivity

Rudolf Steiner calls this exercise a physical exercise in a spiritual way, it is also termed acceptance, tolerance, trust in the environment, the sense for an affirmative view of life, being uninhibited, and observing the beautiful and true in all things.

Often we first look at the reprehensible, contradictory and ugly side of things. In this exercise we should consciously abstain from criticism, and instead develop a stance where we can lovingly empathize with the other person and ask: What makes the person do what he does, or be how he is? Such questions can bring us closer to the essence of the other person, which in turn makes it easier to find a positive side than if we condemn.

To understand this better let us look at a Persian legend about Jesus Christ: Christ, with several of his companions, passes by a decaying dog. While the others turn aside disgusted he speaks with admiration of the beautiful teeth of the cadaver. — The bad and ugly should not stop us humans from looking for the good, the beautiful and the true at the same time. Every shadow also has a sunny side.

Impartiality

We often find that we have a preconceived opinion abut a human being or a thing. The soul attitude of this view is one of feeling shut instead of openness and interest. Rudolf Steiner suggests that the human being, for a certain period of time, should try and let everything or every living being be an opportunity for learning new things. 'One can learn from every draught, from every leaf and from each babble of a small child, if one is willing to take on a point of view that one has not used previously.'[65] One should think the impossible is possible!

For this exercise, open up your soul to situations, thoughts or assertions that seem impossible and think that they are possible.

Harmony and steadfastness

Equanimity is developed in the soul when the previous exercises are consistently practised. This awakens a 'conciliatory basic mood,' shown by growing acceptance and tolerance towards other people. Continue to avoid all complacency and criticism towards the imperfect, instead try to understand them.

Rudolf Steiner summarizes the six exercises in the following way:

> When the five qualities previously mentioned
> have been acquired by the soul, then a sixth one
> appears by itself: an inner balance, a harmony of

the spiritual powers. The human being has to find
something in himself which is like a spiritual centre of gravity, which gives him steadfastness and
security despite everything outside which sways
him back and forth. It is not necessary to stop
living with things, or to stop making experiences
with the world. It is not correct to avoid things
which make you sway here and there, but *despite
this* live life to the full while keeping a firm hold
of inner balance and harmony.[66]

To finish I want to mention the *reflection exercise* mentioned
repeatedly by Rudolf Steiner, which can help us to attain an
objective view of ourselves: in the evening, stand back a little
and look at yourself as if you were a stranger and observe the
happening of the day in reverse order. This can of course be
done in different ways. Here I would like to suggest a theme-
related reflection. This can contain the following questions:

- What kind of noises, sounds, voices etc have I heard today?
  How did I listen today? Who did I listen to particularly well,
  who was I not able to listen to properly?
- What meaningful thing did I say today, what was the situation? How did I intrude on the personality of my child, of
  my partner?
- What did I do today? When did I pay complete attention to
  something, where less?

Please use these examples as suggestions; there are limitless
questions you can ask yourself. You can change the theme of
the reflection daily, but it is also helpful to retain one theme
for a longer period of time. It is important to remember not
to use this exercise to evaluate your day, but to consciously
observe it. This attitude develop its fruits as you proceed with
the exercise.

To end this chapter I would like to give you several verses and poems for inner contemplation. Particularly when you are lacking time a verse can be as helpful as a longer exercise to lift you out of your daily circumstances.

Meditation of peace

I carry rest within me,
I bear within myself
Forces giving me strength.
Full will I fill myself
With the warmth of my forces,
I will drench myself
With the power of my will.
And I will feel
How rest outpours itself
Through all my being,
If I strengthen myself
To come upon rest
As a force within me
Though this my striving's power.

Rudolf Steiner[67]

Voice of the angel

Do not speak to me:
I cannot answer you,
I only hear
The sounds of songs of praise.
I have a task,
Know: to serve the holy songs
Sound by sound.
But have no fear:
Above all words
And all that happens

And has ever happened,
Resounds this sound
Everywhere.
Take heart and join in!
And you will be near to me.

Albrecht Goes

LISTEN, listen! — oh you, my God —
Only deaf ones know what listening does,
And wait in the ice of silence
For your living word.
For human words they too are waiting ...
Hardly their heart dares to arise,
To take to heart an answer,
When once they do feel spoken to,
And joyfully tremble with fright.
But their life — oh you, my God —
Their life is still full of the promise,
That you will enter their flesh as lasting word
And transform the tower of shame to a temple.

Christine Lavant

O Christ,
Grant me the power
That I may govern
Hands, and feet, and senses, and word.
Help me to use them
For right deeds and right ways,
For pure thoughts
And loving counsel.
Lead me,
So that I do not build errors into my being.
Warn me, that I should forgive
When someone has harmed me!

Then I shall build in such a way,
That I will the Good
When I return.
Warn me, that I should repent
When I have caused someone pain.
Then I shall build in such a way
That I shall think the truth
When I return.
Bestow it upon me, that I share the joy
And the sufferings of others,
That I become a fellow creator
In harmony with each one's ways.

Albert Steffen

13. Psychological Distress and the Birth Pangs of the Consciousness Soul

In this chapter I would like to round up the themes concerning 'why children don't listen' by looking at questions of our present time, which are increasingly influenced by the era of the consciousness soul. This era has been developing since the fifteenth century, and we humans (as individuals) of this epoch strongly feel its trials and effects.

We have already heard in Chapter 9 that children are competent to mirror the behaviour of adults, giving us echoes which can help us to regain our own lost competence. In this way we can succeed in casting off our fruitless and unloving deeds and habits.

Children want to have an equal, personal dialogue with adults. But before reaching this stage, many parents and pedagogues need to overcome difficult trials, which helps them to become more conscious in relation to their children.

At this point I think it is helpful to step back from the personal and look towards the universal challenges and phenomena of our time. The lecture given by Rudolf Steiner in 1916 *psychological distress and the birth pangs of the consciousness soul* can help to understand this phenomenon from a spiritual point of view.[68]

In this lecture Rudolf Steiner describes the contrast of the last epoch of culture, the sentient and comprehension soul-era, to the present epoch of culture, in which the consciousness soul needs to be developed. Before the fifteenth century the human being grew up in such a way that his intellect developed with his overall natural potential. It was not necessary to educate the intellect as is increasingly the case nowadays. And the same is true for encounters: when two people met, they knew how to

175

adapt themselves to each other with greater ease than is the case
nowadays.

> In these earlier centuries human beings did not
> pass by one another with as little interest as they
> so often do nowadays. When people meet nowa-
> days it often takes them a long time to get to
> know one another properly. The have to learn all
> kinds of things about each other before mutual
> trust can begin to form. What it takes us a long
> time to achieve, and even there we frequently
> fail, was achieved instantaneously when people
> met one another in former centuries [...]. They
> quickly succeeded in encountering one another
> by virtue of their individuality, without having to
> spend a long time exchanging thoughts and feel-
> ings first.[69]

Nowadays, humanity has become so developed and organized
that the world is encircled by a completely different network of
feeling relationships. A meeting does not have such a 'powerful'
effect that the one person knows immediately who the other
is and what he means, rather as the result of the developing
consciousness soul people feel separated from each other. The
consciousness soul makes the human being much more a single
individual, a hermit, who lives in relative isolation.

Rudolf Steiner goes on to describe that nowadays human
beings bring a great number of experiences and results with
them from former incarnations. These arise unconsciously in
us when we meet other people. Because of this it takes longer
and is more difficult to get to know the other person. To do
this we need to understand the greater relationships stemming
from our different incarnations and gradually allow 'what [we]
have experienced with each other to rise up in [our] feelings,
in [our] instincts.'[70] This can only succeed if the individual finds
the energy for inner development.

'People will find it more and more difficult to
achieve the appropriate relation to each other
[…], because this achieving the appropriate relationship with one another entails the application
of inner development, inner activity. This has
already begun, but it will become more and more
widespread and intense. Even now it is already
difficult for people brought together by karma
to understand one another directly. One reason
is that other karmic connections may be sap-
ping their strength, so that they lack the energy
to bring to the fore instinctively everything they
have in them from earlier incarnations. People are
brought together and love one another; certain
influences from earlier incarnations bring this
about. But it is not only those who meet each
other during the course of life who will have
to try and find out whether what arises within
them can provide sufficient bases for an ongoing
relationship. Sons and daughters, too, will find it
increasingly difficult to understand their mothers and fathers, parents will find it harder and
harder to understand their children, and the same
will be the case for sisters and brothers. Mutual
understanding will become increasingly difficult
because it will be more and more necessary for
people first of all to let what lives in them karmi-
cally emerge properly from the depths of their
being.[71]

According to Rudolf Steiner, we need to clearly see these difficult circumstances in this present era of the consciousness soul,
and not remain dreamily in the dark.

'If humanity […] were not faced with the prospect
of having difficulty in mutual understanding, then

the consciousness soul would be unable to develop.
The consequence of this would be that people
would have to live collectively more on the basis of
natural instincts. The individual aspects of the consciousness soul would be unable to develop; so it is
essential for humanity to undertake this trial.[72]

We as humans need to learn to form our present time more consciously. One of the tasks of Rudolf Steiner's spiritual science is
to contribute towards a more conscious forming in this sense. In
this context Rudolf Steiner gives the remedy for these difficulties
in mutual understanding the term *social understanding*

Spiritual science needs to increasingly develop from an abstract
ideal towards a completely concrete teaching, towards real life. The
basis for social understanding will be a specific kind of knowledge
about the human being – an awakening of human interest. Practical
psychology, practical study of the human soul and practical study of
life will be necessary in future, as this will lead to a real social understanding of human evolution. We need such a study and knowledge
of the human being to correctly understand the emergent, growing
human being — to rightly understand the child, each one developing with their own individuality.

We are far too quick to repeatedly judge other people,
whether as parents, partner, friend or teacher, by letting our
swaying feelings govern us, sticking to preconceived ideas and
compartmentalizing, perhaps without even knowing the other
person adequately. This kind of meeting is still governed by the
character of the sentient soul, which usually leads us to repeated
problems and trials in mutual understanding between people.
This is the point where human beings receive the chance to
practise and develop the qualities of the consciousness soul:

Human beings always have to undergo trials when
such developments are under way, for they are
resisted by the forces of opposition. So feelings of
sympathy and antipathy will become widespread,

> and only in the conscious struggle against super-
> ficial likes and dislikes will the consciousness souls
> be rightly born. [73]

These trials will also affect religious life. In previous times group religions were formed, nowadays religious understanding penetrates directly into the soul of the individual. New forms of understanding Christianity are necessary, as out of itself it does not affect people anymore. It has become necessary to understand other religions and the different aspects of Christ beliefs.

Rudolf Steiner emphasizes the importance of social understanding in the realm of human relationships and freedom of thought in the realm of religion, of religious life. And to develop the consciousness soul the person of our new age requires a third aspect — knowledge of the spirit through spiritual science.

> There are already plenty of people who watch
> with a bleeding heart these situations which,
> though necessary, can only work properly if they
> are rightly understood... the impulse for a new
> way of working in the world must be wrung
> consciously from the heart's blood. The estrange-
> ment of individuals from one another will happen
> of its own accord, but what is to flow from the
> human heart must be consciously sought. [74]

I would like to contribute towards a practical understanding and knowledge of the soul with this book, which ideally would carry the title *it is only with the heart that one can see rightly*. May it prepare the way to the heart and hopefully enable many lights to shine up to him who lovingly stands beside us with a helping hand.

Endnotes

1 Gerald Hüther, *Biologie der Angst. Wie aus Stress Gefühle werden,* (The Biology of fear. How feelings develop out of stress). Göttingen 1997

2 Barbara Denjean-von Stryk, *Sprich, dass ich dich sehe. Die Sprache als Schulungsweg in Kunst, Erziehung und Therapie,* Stuttgart 1996.

3 Ibid.

4 Monika Kiel-Hinrichsen, *Warum Kinder trotzen. Phänomene, Hintergründe und pädagogische Begleitung,* Stuttgart 1999.

5 This phase of life is described in more detail in the following book: Monika Kiel-Hinrichsen / Renate Kviske, *Wackeln die Zähne – wackelt die Seele. Der Zahnwechsel. Ein Handbuch für Eltern und Erziehende,* Stuttgart 2004.

6 Rudolf Steiner, *Die geistig-seelische Grundkräfte der Erziehungskunst, Spirituelle Werte in Erziehung und sozialem Leben* (GA 305), Dornach 1991,

7 This relationship does not remain stable, but only shows continuity around twelve years of age.

8 See Rudolf Steiner, *Geisteswissenschaftliche Gesichtspunkte zur Therapie* (GA 313), Dornach 2001, Lecture from the 14th of April 1921

9 Hermann Koepke, *Das neunte Lebensjahr. Seine Bedeutung in der Entwicklung des Kindes,* Dornach 2002.

10 Ibid.

11 Hans Müller-Wiedemann, *Mitte der Kindheit. Das neunte bis zwölfte Lebensjahr. Beiträge zu einer anthroposophischen Entwicklungspsychologie.* Stuttgart 2003.

12 Jeanne Meijs, *Der schmale Weg zur inneren Freiheit. Ein Leitfaden durch die Zeit der Pubertät,* Stuttgart 2003.

13 Ibid.

14 Ibid.

15 Hans Müller-Wiedemann, *Mitte der Kindheit. Das neunte bis zwölfte Lebensjahr. Beiträge zu einer anthroposophischen Entwicklungspsychologie.* Stuttgart 2003.

16 Rudolf Steiner, *Wahrspruchworte* (GA 40), Dornach 1998, p. 353.

17 See Rudolf Steiner, *Geistige Hierarchien und ihre Widerspiegelung in der physischen Welt Tierkreis, Planeten, Kosmos* (GA 110), Dornach 1991, p. 183

18 Rudolf Steiner/Marie Steiner-von Sivers, *Sprachgestaltung und dramatische Kunst* (GA 282), Dornach 1981, Lecture from the 6th of September 1924, pp. 85.

19 After John O. Stevens, *Die Kunst der Wahrnehmung. Übungen der Gestalttherapie,* Gütersloh 2002.

20 From: Manfred Gührs/Claus Nowak, *Das konstruktive Gespräch. Ein Leitfaden für Beratung, Unterricht und Mitarbeiterführung mit Konzepten der Transaktionsanalyse.* Meezen 2002.

181

21 See Friedemann Schulz von
    Thun, *Miteinander reden,* Volume
    1: *Störungen und Klärungen.*
    Allgemeine Psychologie der
    Kommunikation, Reinbek 2005.
22 Ibid.
23 Reinbek 2005.
24 Gerald Hüther, *Biologie der Angst.*
    Wie aus Stress Gefühle werden,
    Göttingen 1997.
25 See also Thomas A. Harris, *Ich*
    bin o.k., du bist o.k. Wie wir uns
    selbst besser verstehen und unsere
    Einstellung zu anderen verbessern
    können. Eine Einführung in die
    Transaktionsanalyse. Reinbek
    2002, and Rüdiger Rogoll und
    Christa Marwedel, *Ich mag mein*
    Kind – mein Kind mag mich!
    Wie das Leben mit Kindern Spaß
    machen kann. Transaktionsanalyse
    für Eltern, Freiburg i. Br. 1989.
26 Rüdiger Rogoll und Christa
    Marwedel, *Ich mag mein Kind*
    – mein Kind mag mich! Wie das
    Leben mit Kindern Spaß machen
    kann. Transaktionsanalyse für Eltern,
    Freiburg i. Br. 1989.
27 Ibid.
28 Ibid.
29 See Monika Kiel-Hinrichsen,
    Warum Kinder trotzen. Phänomene,
    Hintergründe und pädagogische
    Begleitung, Stuttgart 1999.
30 Rüdiger Rogoll und Christa
    Marwedel, *Ich mag mein Kind*
    – mein Kind mag mich! Wie das
    Leben mit Kindern Spaß machen
    kann. Transaktionsanalyse für Eltern,
    Freiburg i. Br. 1989.
31 Ibid.
32 Ibid.
33 Ibid.
34 Gerald Hüther/Helmut Bonney,
    Neues vom Zappelphilipp, ADS/

    ADHS verstehen, vorbeugen und
    behandeln, Düsseldorf 2002.
35 See Manfred Gührs/Claus Nowak,
    Das konstruktive Gespräch. Ein
    Leitfaden für Beratung, Unterricht und
    Mitarbeiterführung mit Konzepten der
    Transaktionsanalyse, Meezen 2002.
36 Karl König, *Der Kreis der*
    zwölf Sinne und die sieben
    Lebensprozesse, Stuttgart 1999.
37 Michaela Glöckner, *Macht in der*
    zwischenmenschlichen Beziehung.
    Grundlagen einer Erziehung zur
    Konfliktbewältigung, Stuttgart 2001.
38 Karl König, *Der Kreis der*
    zwölf Sinne und die sieben
    Lebensprozesse, Stuttgart 1999.
39 Rudolf Steiner, *Das Rätsel*
    des Menschen, Die Geistigen
    Hintergründe der menschlichen
    Geschichte (GA 107), Dornach
    1978, Lecture from the 2nd of
    September 1916, p. 245.
40 Michaela Glöckner, *Macht in der*
    zwischenmenschlichen Beziehung.
    Grundlagen einer Erziehung zur
    Konfliktbewältigung, Stuttgart 2001.
41 Wolfgang Schad,
    „Sinnesentwicklung und
    Sozialfähigkeit," in: *Erziehungskunst,*
    in booklet 9 (1991).
42 Willi Aeppli, *Sinnesorganismus,*
    Sinnesverlust Sinnespflege. Die
    Sinneslehre Rudolf Steiners in
    ihrer Bedeutung für die Erziehung.
    Stuttgart 1996.
43 Rudolf Steiner on the 25th of
    October 1909.
44 Michaela Glöckner, *Macht in der*
    zwischenmenschlichen Beziehung.
    Grundlagen einer Erziehung zur
    Konfliktbewältigung, Stuttgart
    2001.
45 Ibid.
46 Benita Quadflieg-von Vegesack.

Ungewöhnliche Kleinkinder und ihre heilpädagogischen Förderung. Von der Geburt bis zur Einschulung. Ostfildern/Stuttgart 1998.

47 Gerald Hüther/Helmut Bonney, *Neues vom Zappelphilipp, ADS/ ADHS verstehen, vorbeugen und behandeln,* Düsseldorf 2002.

48 Ibid.

49 *Der Spiegel,* Heft 11 (2002).

50 Rudolf Steiner, *Wahrspruchworte* (GA 40), Dornach 1998, p. 298.

51 Jesper Juul, *Das kompetente Kind. Auf dem Weg zu einer neuen Wertgrundlage für die ganze Familie,* Reinbek 2003.

52 Ibid.

53 Daniel Goleman, *Emotionale Intelligenz, EQ.* Munich 1997.

54 See also Claude Steiner, *Emotionale Kompetenz,* Munich 1999.

55 Abraham H. Maslow, *Motivation und Persönlichkeit,* Reinbek 2002.

56 See also Walter Pachter, *Ich will doch nur das Beste für mein Kind. Spielregeln und Übungen nach Gordons Familienkonferenz.* Freiburg i. Br. 1992.

57 Thomas Gordon, *Familienkonferenz. Die Lösung von Konflikten zwischen Eltern und Kind.* Munich 1999.

58 Walter Pacher, *Ich will doch nur das Beste für mein Kind. Spielregeln und Übungen nach Gordons Familienkonferenz.* Freiburg i. Br. 1992.

59 Thomas Gordon, *Familienkonferenz. Die Lösung von Konflikten zwischen Eltern und Kind.* Munich 1999.

60 Heinz Zimmermann, *Sprechen, Zuhören, Verstehen in Erkenntnis- und Entscheidungsprozessen,*

Stuttgart 1998.

61 Friedemann Schulz von Thun, *Miteinander reden,* Volume 3: *Das „innere Team" und situationsgerechte Kommunikation,* Reinbek 2005.

62 For a more in-depth view, see also Friedemann Schulz von Thun, *Miteinander reden,* Volume 3: *Das „innere Team" und situationsgerechte Kommunikation,* Reinbek 2005.

63 For example: Rudolf Steiner, *Anweisungen für eine esoterische Schulung* (GA 245), Special Edition, Dornach 1999, pp. 15.

64 Florin Lowndes, *Die Belebung des Herzchakra. Ein Leitfaden zu den Nebenübungen Rudolf Steiners,* Stuttgart 2000.

65 Rudolf Steiner, *Die Geheimwissenschaft im Umriss* (GA 13), Dornach 1989, p. 335.

66 Rudolf Steiner, *Die Stufen der höheren Erkenntnis* (GA 12), Dornach 1993, pp. 33.

67 Rudolf Steiner, *Anweisungen für eine Esoterische Schulung* (GA 245), Special Edition, Dornach 1999, p. 80.

68 Rudolf Steiner, „Wie kann die seelische Not der Gegenwart überwunden werden? Soziales Menschenverständnis – Gedankenfreiheit – Geisterkenntnis," in Rudolf Steiner, *Die Verbindung zwischen Lebenden und Toten* (GA 168), Dornach 1995, Single Edition Dornach 1994.

69 Ibid. Dornach 1994, pp. 9,

70 Ibid, p. 12.

71 Ibid, pp. 12.

72 Ibid, p. 13.

73 Ibid, p. 17.

74 Ibid, pp.23.

Bibliography

Anschütz, Marieke, *Children and Their Temperaments,* Floris Books, Edinburgh 1995.

Gordon, Thomas, *Parent Effectiveness Training,* Three Rivers Press, California 2000.

Glöckler, Michaela and Wolfgang Goebel, *A Guide to Child Health,* Floris Books, Edinburgh 2003.

Harris, Thomas A, *I'm OK, You're OK,* Arrow, London 1995 and Harper Paperbacks, New York 2004.

Jaffke, Freya, *Work and Play in Early Childhood,* Floris Books, Edinburgh 1996.

Jenkinson, Sally, *The Genius of Play,* Hawthorn Press, Stroud 2001.

Koepke, Hermann, *Encountering the Self: Transformation and Destiny in the Ninth Year,* Anthroposophic Press, New York 1989.

König, Karl, *The First Three Years of the Child: Walking, Speaking, Thinking,* Floris Books, Edinburgh 2004.

Lievegood, Bernard, *Phases of Childhood: Growing in Body, Soul and Spirit,* Floris Books, Edinburgh 2005.

Oldfield, Lynne, *Free to Learn,* Hawthorn Press, Stroud 2001.

Petrash, Jack. *Understanding Waldorf Education,* Gryphon House, Maryland, 2002 and Floris Books, Edinburgh 2003.

Sleigh, Julian, *Thirteen to Nineteen: Discovering the Light,* Floris Books, Edinburgh 1998.

Steiner, Rudolf, *How to Know Higher Worlds,* Anthroposophic Press, New York 1994.

—, *Speech and Drama,* Anthroposophic Press, New York and Rudolf Steiner Press London 1986.

Freya Jaffke

Work and Play in Early Childhood

Rhythm and repetition, together with example and imitation, are the pillars on which early learning is based. Freya Jaffke applies these simple principles in practical and sensible ways.

She describes children's play in a Steiner-Waldorf kindergarten setting, and provides tried and tested advice on this important stage of development.

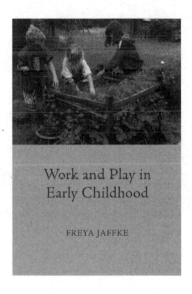

www.florisbooks.co.uk

Bernard C. J. Lievegoed

Phases of Childhood

Growing in Body, Soul and Spirit

Drawing on the educational ideas of Rudolf Steiner, and on a philosophical tradition going back to Goethe and Schiller, Lievegoed turns away from the materialist nineteenth-century notion of 'knowledge is power' which still pervades mainstream education today. He describes the three main stages of child development — pre-school, schoolchild and teenager — in a clear and concise way. Lievegoed shows that each stage of roughly seven years has its own character, and its own genetic and biographical potential.

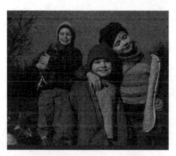

PHASES OF CHILDHOOD

Growing in Body, Soul and Spirit

Bernard C J Lievegoed

www.florisbooks.co.uk

Michaela Glöckler & Wolfgang Goebel

A Guide to Child Health

This book is an acclaimed guide to children's physical, psychological and spiritual development. Combining medical advice with issues of upbringing and education, this is a definitive guide for parents.

Throughout, the book is extremely practical, covering all childhood illnesses, ailments and conditions, and home nursing. The authors also outline the connection between education and healing, with all that this implies for the upbringing and good health of children. Medical, educational and religious questions often overlap, and in the search for the meaning of illness it is necessary to study the child as a whole — as body, soul and spirit.

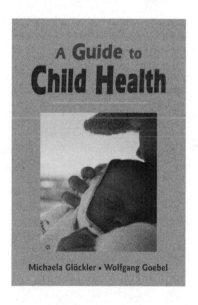

www.florisbooks.co.uk